Balancing the Act

Balancing the Act

The impact of the Children Act 1989 on family link services for children with disabilities

Margaret Macadam and Carol Robinson, Norah Fry Research Centre

The National Children's Bureau was established as a registered charity in 1963. Our purpose is to identify and promote the interests of all children and young people and to improve their status in a diverse society.

We work closely with professionals and policy makers to improve the lives of all children but especially young children, those affected by family instability, children with special needs or disabilities and those suffering the effects of poverty and deprivation.

We collect and disseminate information about children and promote good practice in children's services through research, policy and practice development, publications, seminars, training and an extensive library and information service.

The Bureau works in partnership with Children in Wales and Children in Scotland.

The **Joseph Rowntree Foundation** has supported this project as part of its programme of research and innovative development projects, which it hopes will be of value to policy makers and practitioners. The facts presented and views expressed in this report, however, are those of the authors and not necessarily those of the Foundation.

ISBN 1 874579 69 5 ✓

Published by National Children's Bureau Enterprises, 8 Wakley Street, London EC1V 7QE. Telephone 0171 843 6000.

National Children's Bureau Enterprises is the trading company for the National Children's Bureau (Registered Charity number 258825).

Typeset by Books Unlimited (Nottm), NG19 7QZ.

Printed and bound in the United Kingdom by Redwood Books

Contents

List of tables   vii

List of figures   viii

Acknowledgements   ix

Summary   1

1   Introduction   6

    Background   6
    Aims and objectives   8
    Methods and respondent profiles   9

2   Regulations for children   19

    Child care plans   19
    Visiting the child in placement   23
    Reviews of the child's plan   26
    Medical Assessments   31
    The limit on care   34
    Charging for use of the service   36
    Parents from minority ethnic groups   37
    Discussion   38

3   Regulations for carers   41

    Registration of carers   41
    Reviewing and reapproving carers   42
    Carers' documents   45
    Preparation and training of carers   48
    Recruitment of carers   49
    Carers from minority ethnic groups   50
    Discussion   51

4 Overview   **52**

     Overall effects   52
     The way forward   54

5 Conclusions and recommendations   **56**

Postscript   **61**

References   **63**

Index   **65**

List of tables

1: Geographical spread of sample   12

2: Number of respondents   17

3: Number of years of involvement with the service – percentages in each band   18

4: The child's plan: proportion of children within each service for whom there is a plan of some description   19

5: Proportion of children within each service who are visited by a social worker during their first overnight stay   24

6: The child's plan: frequency of reviews   27

7: Proportion of children within each service for whom a medical report had been obtained before the start of a placement   32

8: The percentage of services where the foster carer approval process was operational, undertaking each of the steps specified   42

List of figures

1a: Service size in terms of numbers of children placed for 24-hour stays   10

1b: Service size in terms of numbers of carers offering 24-hour stays   10

2: Number of reviews in past year according to files   27

3: Allocated days on children's files (Apr. 1992 – Mar. 1993)   35

4: Frequency of carer's review noted on files   43

5: Proportion of services issuing Foster Care Agreements   46

6: Proportion of services issuing Foster Placement Agreements   46

Acknowledgements

We are grateful to Anne Williams for typing this report and for her support throughout the project.

We also wish to thank all those who participated in the research, especially the staff, parents, and carers who took part in the in-depth studies.

Thanks are also due to our Research Advisory Group who guided us through all stages of the study.

This work would not have been possible without the Joseph Rowntree Foundation – we are indebted to them for their support.

The findings from the national survey presented here are substantially drawn from the *Findings* paper published by the Joseph Rowntree Foundation (Robinson and Macadam, 1993).

The authors

Dr. Carol Robinson has been a researcher of short-term care for twelve years. Prior to joining the Norah Fry Research Centre, where she is now a Senior Research Fellow, she was a social worker for Essex County Council. She has published several books and pamphlets on family link services including *Home and Away* (Ventura Press), *Why are we Waiting* and *New Directions* (HMSO), the latter with Dr Kirsten Stalker.

Margaret Macadam is a Research Fellow at the Norah Fry Research Centre, University of Bristol, and has eleven years experience in research and social policy analysis. She is the author of various articles on the themes addressed in this book.

Summary

Background

When the Children Act 1989 came into force in 1991, one of the key areas to be affected was the provision of short-term care in family settings for children with disabilities (family link services). The study reported here was prompted by concerns expressed by practitioners in family link services about the appropriateness and practicalities of the Family Placement Regulations brought in by the Act.

Study aims

The main aim of the study was to assess the extent to which the Family Placement Regulations have been implemented by family link services, to evaluate the impact the regulations have had, and in particular to see whether they improved practice in placing children with disabilities.

Method

The study was carried out two stages. Initially, a postal survey was conducted with all family link services for children in England and Wales. The second stage involved a detailed study of six family link services to see how they were operating under the Children Act. This involved:

- in-depth interviews with staff, parents and link carers;
- an examination of service records;
- a postal survey of parents and carers.

Findings

Child care plans

- Most link services did not have full child care plans as specified by the Children Act for children going to stay over 24 hours with link families.

- The majority of services did have a plan of some description for at least some of their children, but it usually only related to the link placement, rather than providing a full assessment of the child's needs.
- Link staff agreed with the need to have plans but did not have the resources and were not in a position to make full assessments.
- Parents were generally happy with the types of plans that they received.

Recommendation

We recommend that, unless more resources can be found, the requirement for full child care plans be restricted to the heaviest users. A simpler link placement agreement should suffice for other users, at least for the first year, after which a full plan should be drawn up.

Initial visits

- Few services were meeting the Children Act requirement to visit all children during their first overnight stay with a link family.
- Link staff and carers felt that a visit at this point could be intrusive, inappropriate and impractical.
- An early visit by a social worker was seen as important but the required timing of the visit needed to be changed.
- Other forms of contact were made between link staff, carers, children and their parents, including social work visits during the introductory build-up to the first overnight stay.

Recommendation

We welcome the proposed amendment that would allow some discretion in the timing of the first visit to a child in placement. We believe, however, that the proposed limit (within two weeks of the first overnight stay) is too short. We recommend that the first placement visit should take place within three months of the first overnight stay (or within seven overnight stays, whichever is the sooner) and in any case before the first review.

Reviews

- A minority of services were reviewing the child's plan three times per year, every year, as specified by the Children Act Family Placement Regulations.
- It was far more common to hold two reviews per year.
- Most reviews were informal, held at the home of parents or carers and usually attended only by parents, carers and link staff.
- Staff were positive about the requirement to review, as it provided a useful monitoring structure.
- However, staff considered that it was not necessary to review three times per year, especially after the first year and where links were stable. Moreover, resource constraints were cited as a factor in the lower frequency of reviews.
- Most parents liked the idea of having reviews but also did not agree with the required frequency.
- Both staff and parents thought that two reviews per year would be more appropriate.

Recommendation

We welcome the proposal to treat all placements as continuous after the first year so that the requirement to review three times per year every year no longer applies. The proposed requirement to review placements twice a year is likely to be acceptable to practitioners. However, the requirement for a review after four weeks in the first year is questionable, especially if a child has had few overnight stays at this point. We recommend giving social workers more discretion within a time limit so that the first review has to be carried out within three months or seven overnight stays, whichever is the sooner.

Health assessments

- The majority of services were not complying with the Act's requirement to obtain an annual medical report for all children staying overnight with a link family.
- Information on the child's health needs was usually provided by the parents.
- Some staff questioned the appropriateness of this requirement, given that parents updated carers directly with any changes in their child's health and children with complex needs were seen regularly by consultants.

- Most carers reported that they were satisfied with the level of information provided by parents.

Recommendation

We welcome the proposed amendment to this Regulation which removes the requirement to have an annual medical examination and a written assessment of health. We recommend that the new Guidance stresses the importance of regular updates in writing to carers to ensure that drug and treatment information is accurate at all times. These should be verified by the child's GP. This is particularly important for children with complex health care needs or progressive conditions.

Carer registration

- The majority of carers working for family link services were being registered using the fostering approval process, as laid down by the Children Act.
- Most services were complying or intended to comply with the requirement to review and reapprove their carers annually.
- Staff viewed positively the requirement to use foster carer registration. Some had always registered carers in this way.
- Staff also saw the reapproval requirement as good practice.
- Carers accepted that their registration and reapproval was necessary to safeguard the child.
- Some carers welcomed the reapproval process as an opportunity to air their views.
- Parents were generally happy with the required processes which provided extra protection for their children.
- About two thirds of services were issuing relevant documentation to at least some of their carers. These documents outline the services' and the carers' general responsibilities and details of the arrangements for particular children.
- Fewer than half of the services were issuing these documents to *all* of their carers.
- Both carers and staff found the documents useful.

Recommendation

The Regulations regarding carer approval have been applied relatively successfully and have generally been helpful in clarifying the status of carers. We, therefore, recommend that these Regulations remain unchanged.

Conclusions

Family link services are clearly having problems implementing the Regulations brought in by the Children Act. In many services, growth is at a standstill and little time is available for recruiting and supporting carers or making new links. Staff welcomed the Act for its positive contributions. They were keen, however, not to over-formalise their services and in some cases appear to have implemented the Regulations with a 'light touch'. This is reflected in the low level of negative reaction to the Act from parents and carers. The overriding message was that regulations were needed, but that they were unrealistic and unworkable in their present form.

The way forward lies in producing a set of regulations that safe-guard the welfare of the child whilst allowing family link services to flourish. We welcome the proposals contained in the consulta-tion papers issued recently by the Department of Health (DH, 1994b and 1995a) and see them as going some way to reaching this goal. However, we would like to see some attention paid to clarify-ing three other issues.

First, the Family Placement Regulations only apply after a 24-hour stay. Consequently, children could stay away from home overnight after school for up to five nights before the Regulations apply. This situation should be rectified.

Second, clarification is needed of the purpose, timing and allo-cation of responsibility surrounding the writing of child care plans.

Third, there should be a tightening rather than relaxing of the Regulations regarding the 90-day limit on the amount of time a child may spend each year with a carer. It is currently possible for children to spend 90 days in each of a number of settings. If this happens, it is important that there is a clear strategy for monitor-ing and planning to ensure the arrangements protect the child's welfare.

1. Introduction

Background

The Children Act 1989, which came into force on 14 October 1991, has been described as the most radical reform of child care legislation this century. It repeals a total of 55 statutes and has introduced a mass of new guidance and regulations on virtually all aspects of private and public child care. The Act also represents a major landmark in social policy for children with disabilities by including them for the first time in mainstream child care law. This conveys the message that children with disabilities are like other children and should be treated similarly.

Prior to the introduction of the Children Act, children with disabilities were accommodated either in families or in residential homes under the wide provisions of the National Health Service Act of 1977. This allowed for the arrangement of short breaks away from home for children with disabilities without the usual formalities of reception into care or charging. Unfortunately, the lack of formal procedures among service providers for the planning and monitoring of placements meant that children sometimes drifted into long-term care arrangements without any legal protection for their welfare. The Children Act sought to ensure that this protection was afforded to all children accommodated away from home.

The Children Act itself makes few direct references to children with disabilities, other than to classify them as children in need and to define in pejorative terms what is meant by 'disabled'. However, Schedule 2 of the Act does specify that services should 'minimise the effects of children's disabilities upon them'. This places a duty on service providers, not only to help children gain physical independence, but also to develop integrated rather than segregated services. The family link services studied for this research were already offering integrated services to children by placing them with ordinary families in the community who were recruited and trained for the work. In this way, children have the opportunity to mix with non-disabled children and adults and to broaden their horizons, while their parents are able to recharge their batteries.

Following the introduction of the Children Act, family link services for children with disabilities were forced to operate under a completely new legal framework and were subject to the same regulations as other foster placements. This study sought to discover what the true impact of the new Regulations and Guidance on Family Placements would be on family link services.

Family link services

According to Shared Care [UK], there are currently 331 family link schemes in operation in the UK. Of these, 74 are for adults and 257 for children. Most services are run by local authority social services departments, although 21 per cent are run by voluntary agencies (Beckford and Robinson, 1993). Such services are oversubscribed with virtually all of them having a waiting list: the average number of children each service had on its waiting list for a link family in 1992 was 18. Children who present challenging behaviour, need high levels of physical care, or come from minority ethnic groups are most likely to wait for services (Stalker and Robinson, 1991).

The demand for family link services is clear, but provision is patchy and in some areas family link services are not well developed so that families may have little choice but to use some form of residential home or health service unit. The surveys carried out by the Office of Population Censuses and Surveys (OPCS) during the late 1980s estimated that there were 360,000 children with disabilities under 16, of whom 169,000 were in the higher severity levels (categories six to ten on the OPCS scale). The most recent data indicate that fewer than six per cent of these children have access to family-based care (Beckford and Robinson, 1993).

The Children Act makes it explicit that local authorities may charge if they think it is reasonable to do so and in recent years there has been an increase in the number of services that levy a charge to users (seven per cent of schemes in 1992). However, most children's services remain free. Prior to the introduction of the Children Act, most services offered a limited amount of care. For example, 33 per cent offered between four and eight weeks per annum, while 24 per cent offered less than four weeks. The remainder had no fixed limit (Beckford and Robinson, 1993).

Despite the limited availability of care through family link services, families who use them tend to find them highly satisfactory (Robinson and Stalker, 1990). Equivalent services for young non-disabled people who need a break from home are relatively few in number and are a much more recent development.

The study

The decision to undertake a study that would assess the impact of the Children Act on family link services was prompted by concerns that were being voiced by practitioners about the appropriateness and practicalities of the new Regulations, both in the press (Neary, 1991) and in their contact with the Norah Fry Research Centre. Under the Children Act 1989, local authorities are required to provide services that enable children in need, including children with disabilities, to live in their own homes wherever possible, and that minimise the effects of children's disabilities. Given that family link services are a prime example of such support, it seemed important to look closely at the effects of the new Regulations on the staff who have to implement them, as well as on the carers and users whose links are regulated by them.

A series of projects designed to monitor the impact of the Children Act was being commissioned by the Department of Health. However, there was little being done on the provision of short-term care. There are two exceptions to this – work by Aldgate and Bradley was underway to look at the development of a small number of local authority services offering accommodation to non-disabled young people (Aldgate and others, forthcoming). This focused on factors that contribute to the prevention of long-term family breakdown and the characteristics of families for whom short-term breaks are helpful or unhelpful. The second project with the Department of Health backing concerned the quality of residential short term care and day care services to children with disabilities (Robinson and others, 1994). Neither project aimed to provide an overall assessment of the impact of the Family Placement Regulations on family link services.

The Norah Fry Research Centre therefore submitted a proposal to the Joseph Rowntree Foundation to undertake a study which would address this issue. The Foundation agreed to support the research which was to run for two years, starting in July 1992.

Aims and objectives

The main aim of the study was to assess the extent to which the Family Placement Regulations had affected family link services and improved practice in placing children with disabilities. It was envisaged that the study would yield data that could be used by senior policy makers to help decide whether these Regulations are promoting the central principles of the Children Act in these services.

Specific objectives of the study were:

1. To examine how many family link services were operating within the Children Act Regulations.
2. To discover whether the Act had led to increased standardisation in practices between schemes on such matters as:
    i.   the assessment, registration and training of respite carers;
    ii. the plans made for children receiving short-term care;
    iii. charging users.
3. To study the eligibility criteria for receipt of a service to see if these had changed since the implementation of the Act.
4. To assess whether the number of children using family link services had increased or decreased as a result of the new legislation.
5. To obtain the views of service providers concerning the benefits or otherwise of the Regulations for schemes.
6. To interview parents who were involved in family link schemes prior to the implementation of the Act to find out what they thought of the new Regulations.
7. To discover whether link carers' perceptions of their role had changed as a result of the new, more stringent requirements for their approval as foster carers.
8. To evaluate whether children and young people using family link services were more likely to be consulted about potential and actual placements since the advent of the Act.
9. To assess whether the Regulations were having a differential effect on minority ethnic groups and those on low incomes.

It should be noted that the Family Placement Regulations apply only to children who stay away from home for at least 24 hours at a time and to carers who provide short breaks for this length of time (ie day care services are not affected by these regulations). The above aims and objectives were, therefore, only in respect of family link services providing overnight stays.

Methods and respondent profiles

Phase I: The national survey of services

Method

The aim of this phase was the collection of information about the

Figure 1a: Service size in terms of numbers of children placed for 24-hour stays (n = 172)

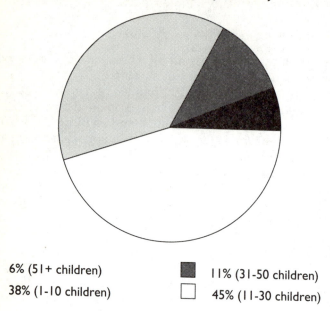

■ 6% (51+ children)	▨ 11% (31-50 children)
▨ 38% (1-10 children)	□ 45% (11-30 children)

Figure 1b: Service size in terms of numbers of carers offering 24-hour stays (n = 172)

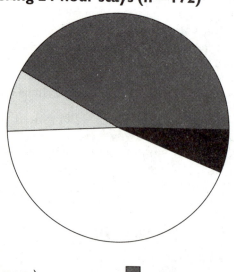

■ 6% (51+ carers)	▨ 42% (11-30 carers)
▨ 9% (31-50 carers)	□ 43% (1-20 carers)

practices of all the known family link services in England and Wales that provided overnight stays for children with disabilities. Questions focused on the way authorities had applied the Children Act Regulations and the way service coordinators perceived their impact on the service.

Names and addresses of services for children with disabilities were obtained from Shared Care[UK] (formerly the National Association for Family Based Respite Care) whose register is housed at the Norah Fry Research Centre. Additional information about new services was gathered through the regional secretaries of Shared Care [UK].

During phase one, data were collected using a postal questionnaire. This was sent out to service coordinators and was followed up by a telephone call if the form had not been returned within a month. This was done for two reasons:

    i.   to ensure that the recipient understood all the questions;
    ii. to increase the likelihood of a high response rate.

Those people who expressed doubts about their ability to return the questionnaire were encouraged to provide the details over the telephone. Queries on returned questionnaires were also clarified through telephone calls. Fieldwork was undertaken between October and December 1992.

Response rate

Originally, 267 postal questionnaires were sent out. It was discovered subsequently that 52 of these were not potential respondents due to the fact that they were no longer/not yet operating a service (21), were not offering overnight stays (15), were being covered by other questionnaires (13) or were no longer offering a service to children (3). From the potential 215 valid questionnaires, 172 were returned – a response rate of 80 per cent.

The response rate within the different regions was broadly similar with most areas returning between 75 and 82 per cent of questionnaires. The exceptions were the below average response rate from the south west (69 per cent) and the above average rate from the south east of England (90 per cent).

Local authority services and those run by voluntary organisations also had similar response rates (81 per cent and 83 per cent respectively).

Service characteristics

The majority (84 per cent) of services in the sample were run by local authorities. The remainder were mainly run by voluntary organisations (14 per cent) with a few being run jointly (two per cent).

The regional breakdown of respondents' services was as follows:

Table 1:   Geographical spread of sample

Region	% all respondents (n = 172)
Wales	8
Northern	21
Midlands	13
Eastern	6
South east	15
London	9
South	15
South west	13
Total	100

The size of services can be described in terms of both the number of children who are placed and the number of carers who provide overnight stays. As Figure 1a (page 10) shows, the majority of services had up to 30 children on their books, with larger services were in a minority.

Phase 2: Selected services for 'in-depth' analysis

Methods

This phase involved a more detailed look at the operation of six family link services under the Children Act. The six services were selected to reflect the involvement of both local authority and voluntary organisations in the provision of short-term breaks. Other factors that were taken into consideration included:

- size (numbers of children using the service);
- geographical location;
- type of registration used for carers;
- charging/non-charging for the service;
- rural/urban services;
- where local authority services were located (that is, in which part of the social services department);
- areas with minority ethnic populations;
- areas of deprivation.

Data were collected from the six participating services between

June 1993 and January 1994. A seventh service was also approached to take part in a pilot study, during which all research tools were tested prior to their use in the main fieldwork.

Phase two encompassed a number of distinct parts designed to allow a comparison of:

i.   the views of all concerned parties within a single service; and
ii. the different practices and interpretations of the Regulations that may occur among services.

Records search

This was conducted in each service to find out:

i.   whether the number and characteristics of children using the service were different pre- and post-implementation of the Children Act;
ii.   the eligibility criteria before and after the implementation of the Act;
iii. what formal documentation was made concerning the assessment and approval of carers;
iv.   whether child care plans were available for all users;
v.   how far children's views were recorded from assessments and reviews of placements;
vi.   the policy regarding charges.

This exercise provided information about the degree of standardisation in practice among services in relation to the specific Regulations. It also contributed to the overall assessment of the extent to which the Act had been implemented after approximately two years.

Interviews with service providers

Service coordinators and social workers in services were interviewed either individually or in pairs to find out in more detail their views of the Family Placement Regulations. Interviews lasted for between one and one and a half hours. In Area 3 (Northern service), two additional interviews were conducted with children's social workers who were not involved with running the placement service. At this particular service, the link staff were not responsible for individual children and it was therefore thought necessary to talk to the social workers who were responsible for implementing the Regulations as they applied to the children.

Particular attention was paid to whether the stated intentions of the Children Act were being fulfilled and to what extent non-implementation of the Regulations related to a lack of resources, unwillingness to change or a critical assessment of their appropriateness for family-based short-term care. It was acknowledged that these interviews would yield purely subjective views, but they were seen as a valuable way of gaining an understanding of factors that workers in services regard as likely to impede or progress implementation of the principles of the Children Act.

Interviews with parents and carers

A random selection was made from lists of parents and carers who had been involved with each of the six services for at least one year (wherever possible). Roughly twice as many names as were necessary were selected to allow for non-participation. In areas with minority ethnic populations, specific parents and carers were selected to ensure that sufficient numbers were represented in the sample.

A letter was sent to the parents and carers explaining the research and asking if they would be willing to attend a small group discussion. They were then contacted by telephone and where possible recruited for one of the group discussions. The aim was to interview 12 parents and 12 carers in each of the six areas.

The use of groups for interviews with parents and carers was proposed for purely practical reasons. It is acknowledged that some people may be less willing to speak in a group setting than if interviewed separately. The volume of work involved, however, in seeing 72 parents and the same number of carers on an individual basis was regarded as prohibitive, given all the other aspects of the project.

Attendance at the groups was not as high as had been hoped. A number of interviews were therefore conducted individually at the house of the parent or carer, or by telephone. Interviews with non-English speakers were conducted at the homes of these individuals by an interviewer who could speak their language. Individual interviews lasted for about half an hour. Group interviews lasted from 45 minutes to one hour.

Parents and carers were asked to consider a series of questions relating to the impact of the Regulations on the service which they were using or for which they were working. Interviews were tape-recorded and analysed qualitatively. It was decided that quantitative data (such as the number of review meetings attended, the documents received) would be better obtained separately. To this end, a short postal questionnaire was sent with the original letter requesting parents and carers to participate.

Service characteristics

The characteristics of the six selected services were as follows:

Area 1: South Coast service	Small voluntary sector service covering a rural area on the south coast of England (16 children placed for overnight stays).
Area 2: South West service	Medium-sized service based in social services department covering a rural area in the south west of England (28 children placed for overnight stays).
Area 3: Northern service	Large service based in social services department covering a large city in the north of England (124 children placed for overnight stays).
Area 4: Welsh service	Medium-sized service based in social services department covering a small town and surrounding rural area in North Wales (28 children placed for overnight stays).
Area 5: Midlands service	Large voluntary sector service covering an urban area in the West Midlands (60 children placed for overnight stays).
Area 6: London service	Large service based in social services department in a London borough which also encompasses an area of deprivation (50 children placed for overnight stays).

Although we were aiming for a broad spread of sizes, we needed to include services where sufficient numbers of parents and carers would be available, allowing for the likelihood that not all of them would be willing or able to participate in the research. The number of smaller services in this sample, therefore, under-represented the corresponding proportion of such services in the national survey.

The two voluntary sector services were both providing services on behalf of the local authority in the area. One had a service level agreement, the other had joint funding. Three of the four local authority services were managed by children's or children and families' services. One of these was managed through Fostering and Adoption and another was part of a community team, funded by the All Wales Strategy. The fourth local authority service was part of Adult Services, managed by the specialist team for people with learning difficulties.

In the Northern service (Area 3) link staff were responsible only for the carers working for them. All children had allocated social workers from outside the link service who were responsible for implementing all the Family Placement Regulations, as they applied to the child. In the other five areas, staff had responsibility for both children and carers. Although in some cases children had allocated social workers from outside the service, the majority of the workload in relation to the children's regulations was being undertaken by the link social workers. The implications of this situation will become clear in the following chapters.

In two local authority areas, responsibility regarding the children was being redefined at the time of the fieldwork visit. Both these areas were going to move towards a clearer purchaser/provider split. One of them was in the process of negotiating a service level agreement with the district offices of the social services department.

In all six areas, relationships with other agencies were reported as generally being good. Four services had connections with, or were part of, community teams and therefore had particularly effective relationships with health and other social services staff. Most services were in direct contact with special schools and other education staff. On the whole, communication was positive, although one area mentioned a few problems with the re-routing of school transport to carers' homes when children stayed with them during the week.

Children using the service

All services catered for children aged from 0-18/19 years with learning difficulties. Five of the six services also included children with physical disabilities in their eligibility criteria, and two offered a service to children with sensory impairments. The eligibility criteria had changed in only one service since the introduction of the Children Act, to include children under two years old and children with sensory impairments.

For the three areas serving a minority ethnic population, the proportion of service users from these groups were ten per cent, 25 per cent and 50 per cent respectively. It is interesting to compare these figures with the corresponding profile of carers working for these three services. In each area the proportion of carers from minority ethnic groups was lower than that of the children (eight per cent, 20 per cent and 29 per cent respectively). This is in keeping with a national survey which highlighted the dearth of carers from minority ethnic groups (Beckford and Robinson, 1993). Recruitment issues will be discussed in Chapter 4 below.

Respondents: parents and carers

The final totals of parents and carers who returned questionnaires, participated in interviews and whose files (or children's files) were examined, are shown in Table 2 below.

Table 2:   Number of respondents

	Number of parents	Number of carers
Returning questionnaires	70	74
Taking part in interviews	66	69
Whose files or children's files were examined	105	90

It was not possible to match these samples exactly. There was, however, a large degree of similarity. For the majority of the parents and carers who participated in interviews, data from the questionnaires and the records search were available. For most parents and carers who returned questionnaires, data from the records searches were also available.

Table 3 indicates that data from the questionnaires returned and files examined show a broad spread as regards the length of time for which parents and carers had been involved with the service.

Table 3:   Number of years of involvement with the service – percentages in each band

	Parents (source: postal survey) (n = 70) %	Children (source: records) (n = 105) %	Carers (source: postal survey) (n = 74) %	Carers (source: records) (n = 90) %
Up to 1 year	4	18	8	13
1 – 2 years	30	25	16	26
2 – 5 years	31	25	43	43
5 – 10 years	26	30	28	17
10 years +	9	2	4	1
Total	100	100	99*	100

*Due to rounding down

udes to plans

...at the six services thought that the requirement for a child ...a was a good one. The plan was seen as a useful frame-...ich in many cases was consolidating previous good prac-...which would prevent drift for the minority of very heavy ...he service. For example:

...always had plans of a sort, but it's formalised it, recorded it, it's ...s think, made us write it down and date it.'

..., the workload associated with developing plans took its ...example, in the Welsh service the need to draw up 30 ...once had meant that all other work (such as recruiting ...rs and making new links) had ceased.

...aff in the six services visited felt that it was not possible ...to draw up a full child care plan which detailed arrange-...health and education and other short-term care services. ...m not having the resources to do so, it was not felt to be ...te for a provider of one service to make such assess-...ven where children did have separate social workers, this ...uarantee a full plan, as these workers were likely to have ...orities (for example, child protection work). Two areas ...ing away from direct referral systems, so that in order to ...ervice, children would in future have to have a separate ...nt by a key worker/social worker who was not involved in ...ervice. It was thought that this might lead to fuller plans. ...aff felt that they had sufficient contact, albeit informal, ...r professionals and that they would therefore be aware ...ge of other services and any problems they might have. ...evidence from previous research suggests that this con-...not necessarily warranted (Robinson and Stalker, 1991).

ws about plans

...hole, staff appeared to have implemented the planning ...nt with a 'light touch'. This is reflected in parents' views, ...om had strong negative views about plans.

...wo thirds of parents' comments regarding plans were ...tive. The main reason behind the positive attitudes to ...that parents felt that they knew where they stood if ...g was in writing. The indifferent responses (about one ...mments) mainly arose from a feeling that plans were ...ry, as respondents had developed very good relation-...carers and arrangements were made on a friendly

2. Regulations for children

Child care plans

Who had a plan?

The Family Placement Regulations require every child who is to be 'accommodated' (that is, placed for 24 hours or more) under the new legislation to have a child care plan detailing the purpose of the placement as well as information about arrangements for the child's health and education.

As Table 4 shows, the majority of services taking part in the national survey had plans of some description for at least some of their children. Twenty-seven services (16 per cent of the sample) however, had no plans for any of their children. Overall, there was no plan at all for about one third of the children using the services covered by this survey.

Table 4: The child's plan: proportion of children within each service for whom there is a plan of some description

	% services(n = 172)
Plan for all children	38
Plan for some children	46
Plan for no children	16

In the six services visited, almost all the children (95 per cent) whose files were examined had a plan of some description in place. In the Welsh service, the number of plans had risen from none at the time of the survey, to 100 per cent by the time of the visit. Two further areas appeared to have more plans in place than they had noted during the national survey (75 per cent of children using these two services had plans at the time of the survey, rising to just under 100 per cent at the time of the fieldwork visit).

What type of plan was being drawn up?

The national survey revealed that only a minority of children using link services had a full child care plan as specified in the Children Act (21 per cent of all services were using this type of plan). Given that a third of service coordinators were drawing up plans with no other local authority input, it is not surprising that they were often not as detailed as the Act intended.

Forty-eight per cent of respondents in the national survey were using simpler plans, just detailing arrangements for the link placement. Forty per cent of social workers had combined a simple plan for the link placement with the Foster Placement Agreement, which is intended to inform foster carers about individual children.

In the six services visited, the vast majority (87 per cent) of all examined plans referred to link placement arrangements only. In the Northern service, where all children had a separate social worker, only half of the files examined had a full child care plan in place. Most were fairly brief, usually including the following information:

- plan of placement;
- frequency/duration of stays;
- transport arrangements;
- agreement to attend introductory visits and reviews.

In most of the six areas there was little (if anything) to differentiate the plans from the Foster Placement Agreements (where these existed). The majority of plans (80 per cent) were drawn up by link service staff. The remainder were drawn up by the child's social worker/key worker. In the Northern service the children's social workers were responsible for doing this because link service staff had no responsibilities for individual children's plans.

Who was consulted?

In the national survey, 70 per cent of respondents said that the child was consulted when a plan was drawn up. Within this group, however, 16 per cent said that this was only the case for *some* children.

In the six services visited, it appears that parents had been consulted regarding the planned placement in almost all cases (97 per cent). This accords with findings from the parents' questionnaires where 93 per cent said that they were involved in decisions regarding the placement. There was little evidence on the files to show that children had been consulted at the planning stage.

According to the files examined in the six services, copies of a

---

plan had been sent to 81 per cent of parents. than the corresponding results from the qu per cent of parents thought that they had group discussions some parents said they they had received a plan, or were not sure if the paperwork which they had received. T difference in the two figures. Only one third questionnaires from the Northern servic received plans.

Why were plans not issued to all children?

The national survey respondents did not r the concept of planning in principle. The r not having a child care plan of some kind services were:

i. a lack of allocated social worker for organisers were struggling to impl for both the link carers and the chil tance of a caseworker allocated to t

ii. a general lack of resources;

iii. where children did have allocated these individuals had not had tin requested.

Other factors also affected the developmer

Size – only nine per cent of large schemes to 27 per cent of services with fewer than

The type of agency – 96 per cent of volun developing plans for at least some of thei 83 per cent of local authority services. Hc untary organisations (eight per cent) d plans, compared to 23 per cent of local au

The survey showed that about half of services did not have a social worker outs means that there is often a problem about for drafting the child's plan and monitorir theless, the figure compares favourably second Shared Care[UK] survey (Beckfor where over two thirds of children did n workers.

Staff at

All sta
care pl
work, v
tice an
users o

'We'v
made

Howeve
toll. Fo
plans a
new car

Most
for ther
ments f
Apart fi
appropr
ments. I
did not
other pi
were mc
use the
assessm
the link

Some
with oth
of any u
Howeve
fidence i

Parents' v

On the v
requirem
few of wl

About
fairly po:
plans wa
everythii
third of
unnecess
ships wit

2. Regulations for children

Child care plans

Who had a plan?

The Family Placement Regulations require every child who is to be 'accommodated' (that is, placed for 24 hours or more) under the new legislation to have a child care plan detailing the purpose of the placement as well as information about arrangements for the child's health and education.

As Table 4 shows, the majority of services taking part in the national survey had plans of some description for at least some of their children. Twenty-seven services (16 per cent of the sample) however, had no plans for any of their children. Overall, there was no plan at all for about one third of the children using the services covered by this survey.

Table 4: The child's plan: proportion of children within each service for whom there is a plan of some description

	% services(n = 172)
Plan for all children	38
Plan for some children	46
Plan for no children	16

In the six services visited, almost all the children (95 per cent) whose files were examined had a plan of some description in place. In the Welsh service, the number of plans had risen from none at the time of the survey, to 100 per cent by the time of the visit. Two further areas appeared to have more plans in place than they had noted during the national survey (75 per cent of children using these two services had plans at the time of the survey, rising to just under 100 per cent at the time of the fieldwork visit).

What type of plan was being drawn up?

The national survey revealed that only a minority of children using link services had a full child care plan as specified in the Children Act (21 per cent of all services were using this type of plan). Given that a third of service coordinators were drawing up plans with no other local authority input, it is not surprising that they were often not as detailed as the Act intended.

Forty-eight per cent of respondents in the national survey were using simpler plans, just detailing arrangements for the link placement. Forty per cent of social workers had combined a simple plan for the link placement with the Foster Placement Agreement, which is intended to inform foster carers about individual children.

In the six services visited, the vast majority (87 per cent) of all examined plans referred to link placement arrangements only. In the Northern service, where all children had a separate social worker, only half of the files examined had a full child care plan in place. Most were fairly brief, usually including the following information:

- plan of placement;
- frequency/duration of stays;
- transport arrangements;
- agreement to attend introductory visits and reviews.

In most of the six areas there was little (if anything) to differentiate the plans from the Foster Placement Agreements (where these existed). The majority of plans (80 per cent) were drawn up by link service staff. The remainder were drawn up by the child's social worker/key worker. In the Northern service the children's social workers were responsible for doing this because link service staff had no responsibilities for individual children's plans.

Who was consulted?

In the national survey, 70 per cent of respondents said that the child was consulted when a plan was drawn up. Within this group, however, 16 per cent said that this was only the case for *some* children.

In the six services visited, it appears that parents had been consulted regarding the planned placement in almost all cases (97 per cent). This accords with findings from the parents' questionnaires where 93 per cent said that they were involved in decisions regarding the placement. There was little evidence on the files to show that children had been consulted at the planning stage.

According to the files examined in the six services, copies of a plan had been sent to 81 per cent of parents. This is slightly higher than the corresponding results from the questionnaire, where 69 per cent of parents thought that they had received plans. In the group discussions some parents said they could not remember if they had received a plan, or were not sure if the plan was amongst the paperwork which they had received. This could explain the difference in the two figures. Only one third of parents returning questionnaires from the Northern service thought they had received plans.

Why were plans not issued to all children?

The national survey respondents did not report any objections to the concept of planning in principle. The main reasons given for not having a child care plan of some kind for all children using services were:

i.   a lack of allocated social worker for the child: many service organisers were struggling to implement the Regulations for both the link carers and the children without the assistance of a caseworker allocated to the child;

ii.   a general lack of resources;

iii. where children did have allocated social workers, many of these individuals had not had time to develop plans as requested.

Other factors also affected the development of child care plans:

Size – only nine per cent of large schemes had no plans, compared to 27 per cent of services with fewer than ten users.

The type of agency – 96 per cent of voluntary organisations were developing plans for at least some of their children, compared to 83 per cent of local authority services. However, fewer of the voluntary organisations (eight per cent) developed full child care plans, compared to 23 per cent of local authority services.

The survey showed that about half of the children using the services did not have a social worker outside the link service. This means that there is often a problem about where responsibility lies for drafting the child's plan and monitoring the placement. Nevertheless, the figure compares favourably with the finding in the second Shared Care[UK] survey (Beckford and Robinson, 1993) where over two thirds of children did not have separate social workers.

Staff attitudes to plans

All staff at the six services thought that the requirement for a child care plan was a good one. The plan was seen as a useful framework, which in many cases was consolidating previous good practice and which would prevent drift for the minority of very heavy users of the service. For example:

'We've always had plans of a sort, but it's formalised it, recorded it, it's made us think, made us write it down and date it.'

However, the workload associated with developing plans took its toll. For example, in the Welsh service the need to draw up 30 plans at once had meant that all other work (such as recruiting new carers and making new links) had ceased.

Most staff in the six services visited felt that it was not possible for them to draw up a full child care plan which detailed arrangements for health and education and other short-term care services. Apart from not having the resources to do so, it was not felt to be appropriate for a provider of one service to make such assessments. Even where children did have separate social workers, this did not guarantee a full plan, as these workers were likely to have other priorities (for example, child protection work). Two areas were moving away from direct referral systems, so that in order to use the service, children would in future have to have a separate assessment by a key worker/social worker who was not involved in the link service. It was thought that this might lead to fuller plans.

Some staff felt that they had sufficient contact, albeit informal, with other professionals and that they would therefore be aware of any usage of other services and any problems they might have. However, evidence from previous research suggests that this confidence is not necessarily warranted (Robinson and Stalker, 1991).

Parents' views about plans

On the whole, staff appeared to have implemented the planning requirement with a 'light touch'. This is reflected in parents' views, few of whom had strong negative views about plans.

About two thirds of parents' comments regarding plans were fairly positive. The main reason behind the positive attitudes to plans was that parents felt that they knew where they stood if everything was in writing. The indifferent responses (about one third of comments) mainly arose from a feeling that plans were unnecessary, as respondents had developed very good relationships with carers and arrangements were made on a friendly basis. Some parents, although positive about the notion of plans personally, made little use of them. For example:

> 'I have a good host family. They're very flexible so the plan doesn't apply to me really. I think it's a good thing – it lets you know what's going on, you have some guidelines. But I don't refer to it. It goes in the drawer with the other papers.'

The minority of negative comments (fewer than one in six) related to excessive paperwork, inappropriate references to fostering, and excessive rigidity.

Although we were not testing parents and carers about their knowledge of the Children Act, it is worth bearing in mind the extent to which these respondents felt they had been informed about the relevant issues.

Just over one quarter of parents interviewed said that they had not been told anything about the Children Act, or could not remember if they had. A further one third of parents said that they had received some information on this subject but could not remember what they had been told. This contrasts with the corresponding figures from the carers' interviews, where more than 90 per cent said they had been given information about the Children Act. Only four of those who had received information said that they could not remember anything of what they had been told.

For both groups of respondents, the main sources of information were the link staff who had given verbal explanations in most cases. Other sources included specific talks/training sessions (for carers) and leaflets or other written information.

Visiting the child in placement

How many children were visited?

The Children Act specifies that social workers should visit a child at certain intervals during the series of stays with the same carer in any one year. Social workers should visit once during the first stay of 24 hours or more, and again at no more than six monthly intervals in order to monitor the placement. According to the national survey, only one fifth of children had an initial visit during their first 24-hour stay with a link family.

Table 5 (page 24) shows a substantial proportion (over half) of services where none of the children had been visited during the first overnight stay. Only eight per cent of services stated that all children had been visited at this point.

Only 23 per cent of workers claimed to be able to undertake subsequent visits as often as required by the Children Act.

Table 5:　Proportion of children within each service who are visited by a social worker during their first overnight stay

	% local authority	% voluntary organisations	% all services (n = 172)
All children are visited	6	21	8
Some children are visited	33	50	36
No children are visited	61	29	56
Total	100	100	100

The findings from the national survey noted above are backed up by further evidence from children's files. Visits during the child's first overnight stay had only been recorded on ten per cent of the files examined. Obviously the first overnight stay for some links had taken place before implementation of the Children Act. The Regulations, however, still require on-going visits: twice a year every year. Even fewer files (seven per cent) had notes of subsequent visits.

It is possible, however, that children had been seen in placement during the year, but that this had not been noted down. Findings from the carers' questionnaire would seem to suggest this: about half of the sample stated that a social worker had visited them when the child was present at least once (and up to three times) during the previous year. Data are not available on this subject from the carers' files. It could be surmised, however, that at least some of the social worker visits were for other purposes, and the child's presence was coincidental. This might explain why such visits were not noted on the child's file.

Why were visits not being undertaken in line with the Act?

According to the national survey, the likelihood of initial visits was influenced by:

i.　the shortage of out-of-hours resources, which made it difficult to cope with making visits at weekends, when most first overnight stays by children take place (40 per cent);

ii.　the view of many professionals that a visit so early in a placement was either too intrusive, insensitive or overwhelming for the child and the family (30 per cent);

iii.　a general lack of resources (30 per cent);

iv.　the presence of other forms of contact than those specified in the Family Placement Regulations. Many respondents thought these more appropriate (for example visiting the child during the series of short introductory stays which frequently preceded the first overnight stay, or visiting within a certain length of time after the first overnight stay) (20 per cent);

v. the nature of the agency running the service – voluntary organisations were carrying out more initial visits than local authorities (as shown in Table 5 opposite).

There was little resistance to the requirement for subsequent visits. Virtually all national survey respondents who were not implementing it, however, cited resource constraints as the main barrier, including the absence of allocated social workers and the limited amount of out-of-hours resources.

Staff in the six services visited did not, in principle, dispute the need to visit children in the early stages of the placement but many questioned the appropriateness and practicality of the required timing of this visit, largely for the same reasons as outlined above. Staff mentioned that the majority of children have a gradual build-up to their first overnight stay, giving all parties the opportunity to pull out if there are concerns. There was also regular telephone contact in the early stages. In this context, the required early visit was not seen to be essential. Staff could understand the Regulation in the context of emergency foster placements, which would have no introductory stages, but wondered about the reasoning behind it in the context of their service. Alternative suggestions included visiting within a period of six to eight weeks after the first stay. Visits at other times in the year were generally seen as a good thing, although resource constraints still applied.

Carers' attitudes to visits by social workers

Carers were also unhappy about the visiting requirements. Critical comments outnumbered positive ones by about three to one. About half of the objections were connected with the requirement for social workers to visit during the first overnight stay. Carers commented that this would be unsettling for the child and off-putting for themselves. As one carer commented:

> 'It's bad enough for the child, being in a strange house. They might have met you a few times, but to have someone else there as well...'

A few carers wondered whether the visit was necessary, given the length of the approval process and then a gradual series of introductions with the child. Practicalities were also mentioned, with a few carers pointing out that the child's first overnight stay might have to be delayed until a social worker was available, which might not be in the best interests of the child.

The remaining half of the critical comments related to visiting at other times. These were fairly evenly divided between thoughts on the appropriateness of the requirement and the practicalities involved. Carers could not understand the purpose of the visit, commenting that in any case, there was plenty of contact between the link social workers, the parents and themselves and that the parents would soon pick up on any problems. On the practical side, if the visit was unannounced, they might well be out with the child, or the child might not be there (arrangements are often made directly between parents and carers so social workers might not know when the child is coming to stay). If social workers' visits had to be pre-arranged, carers were even less convinced of their usefulness.

Positive comments were fairly evenly split between the view that the visit would be beneficial to the child and an acceptance that if it had to be done, then they would not mind.

Reviews of the child's plan

How often did reviews take place?

The Family Placement Regulations specify that reviews should be conducted three times a year, every year, at intervals of four weeks, three months and six months. This requirement only relates to 'respite' placements; other longer-term placements are subject to two reviews per year after the first year. Only a quarter of coordinators in the national survey reported that this annual requirement was being met. In some of these cases, this was only in the first year and subsequently reviews would take place less often.

As Table 6 shows, the percentage carrying out no reviews at all (22 per cent) compares unfavourably with the situation before the introduction if the Children Act: figures collected between 1989 and 1990 by Shared Care^{UK}, indicated that only 16 per cent of services were *not* doing any such reviews at that time (Orlik and others 1991).

In the six services visited, no reviews had been recorded in the past year for 23 per cent of the children whose files were examined. This figure of 23 per cent is slightly higher than the proportion of parents who reported in the questionnaires that they had not attended any reviews in the last year (15 per cent). In the Northern service, almost half of the files examined had no reviews noted. The questionnaires returned by parents using the Northern service confirm this: nearly half of them had not attended a review in the last year and most of them claimed not to have been invited to attend either.

Table 6:   The child's plan: frequency of reviews

	1990 % services (n = 192)	1992 % services (n = 172)
3 per year	10	15
3 per year in year 1 (less often thereafter)	–	9
2 per year	39	23
1 per year	37	16
Other/varies	–	15
None	16	*22

*This figure includes 14% of respondents who had no plans for any children using their service.

As Figure 2 shows, the most common review frequency noted at the six services was twice per year. Reviews had taken place three times per year in only 13 per cent of cases. In a few cases, children had been with the service for less than a year and so would not have been due for the full number of reviews.

Figure 2:   Number of reviews in past year, according to files (n = 105)

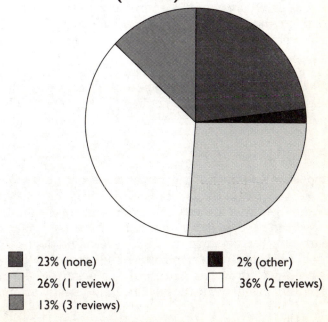

23% (none)   2% (other)
26% (1 review)   36% (2 reviews)
13% (3 reviews)

Half of the cases where reviews were taking place at the required frequency were from the South Coast service which had developed a policy to review at these intervals. Other areas reviewed less frequently unless a review was deemed necessary for some specific reason.

Why are reviewing frequencies not in line with the Children Act?

As with planning, there is no evidence to suggest that coordinators in the national survey were unhappy about the concept of reviewing. They did voice concerns, however, about the frequency of reviews. Thirty-seven per cent of services cited **insufficient resources** as affecting review frequency, while 22 per cent thought that for well-established links, **three reviews per year was excessive and unnecessary**, particularly if the child only stayed away from home a few times per year.

Staff in the six services also viewed positively the requirement to review. It was seen as good practice, providing a useful structure for monitoring the link. For example:

> 'It's essential to have a review structure and I think most families would agree with that. I've always insisted that we meet if only to acknowledge that things are going OK, because you can drift into things not being fine without people realising it.'

The majority disagreed, however, with the requirement to review link placement arrangements three times per year every year for much the same reasons as given in the national survey.

As seen above, the most common reviewing frequency in the six services was twice a year. Staff thought that this was sufficient as long as there was the opportunity for any party to call further reviews as required. Most staff were in regular contact with parents and carers by telephone and so felt that the link was being monitored informally anyway.

What form does the review take?

There is evidence to suggest that reviews are not always being conducted as the Regulations intended. Nearly a quarter of respondents in the national survey stated that at least some of the reviews were conducted on paper only, without holding a meeting. Furthermore, only just over one third of services said that a senior person was present to chair the meeting, as required by the Act. Children's presence at reviews was by no means universal. Forty-two per cent of respondents said that the child usually attended, while a further 17 per cent said that this was only sometimes the case, if thought to be appropriate.

In the six services visited, parents attended almost all reviews (94 per cent) and in 86 per cent of reviews, carers also attended. In the Midlands, the review was held in two parts, one with the parent and one with the carer at their respective homes. Overall, an independent or senior person had attended at least one review in the past year in only 15 per cent of cases where reviews were held.

According to the files examined in the six services, only one quarter of the children had attended at least one review in the last year. In nearly three quarters of reviews, however, it appeared that the views or wishes of the child had been asked for and/or their reactions to placements noted. In 91 per cent of cases where reviews were held, parents were notified of review outcomes. A similar figure emerged from parents' questionnaires, where 85 per cent said that this was the case.

Most reviews at the six services were fairly informal, held either at the parents' or carers' houses. Nevertheless, the content of the review followed a specific format, covering such issues as:

- effects of placement on child/family/carer;
- child's views/reactions;
- changes in circumstances (including health issues);
- whether any changes were required.

Staff views on the nature of reviews

Staff at the six services were concerned to handle reviews sensitively, ensuring that parents did not feel overwhelmed or that they were being regulated. In this context, the presence of a senior person could make the reviews too formal. Staff did not think that the presence of such a person was necessary at all reviews unless there were specific concerns. It was also thought unlikely that a senior person would have time to attend all reviews.

Some staff thought that reviews that involved other agencies (for example, health or education) were not necessary for all children, unless there were particular concerns or usage was particularly high. The majority of staff raised concerns about the practicalities of such reviews. It would be difficult from a resource point of view to get everybody together, especially if there was no keyworker for the child and if this had to happen three times per year for each child.

Although most children did not often attend review meetings, staff thought that it was very important to gauge the child's reactions to the link placement. Some were keen to develop alternative means of involving children:

> 'Clearly there needs to be a lot more thought put into self-advocacy, to devise some means of drawing from the child.'

Parents' and carers' attitudes towards reviews

Amongst parents, there was a fairly even division between positive attitudes and indifference towards reviews, with a small minority of negative attitudes. On the positive side, parents welcomed the opportunity to air their views at review meetings and saw these as a useful way of monitoring any changes in the situation. Parents who were indifferent to reviews mentioned that they had good relationships with their link carers and felt able to raise issues directly with them:

> 'If you can't talk to your host family, you've got a problem.'

They also felt that there was always someone available at the link service if they needed to discuss anything with staff.

On the negative side, a few parents thought that reviews were a waste of time, especially if nothing had changed.

The majority (80 per cent) thought that the required frequency of three reviews per year was too high. Reasons given included the following:

- the money spent on reviews could be better spent on providing more care;
- so many reviews would generate too much paperwork;
- such frequent reviews would often be going over similar ground.

As one parent put it:

> 'You spend all your time going to meetings and filling in forms. If they just rang me up and asked if everything was OK, it would be better.'

Two reviews per year were seen as more appropriate, with the facility to call for extras if the need arose.

On the whole, most parents felt able to say what they wanted to at review meetings. There could be an element of awkwardness for some parents, however, who did not want to upset the carers and risk losing something that was so important to them.

Only a quarter of parents felt able to comment about review meetings at which all relevant agencies are represented. Opinion amongst them was evenly divided between those in favour and those against such meetings. On the positive side, joint meetings could avoid repetition; on the negative side, parents felt that they saw enough professionals anyway and that their presence would not add anything to reviews.

Carers also thought that three reviews per year was too many: for many carers, there was good contact anyway with parents and link staff, and for well-established links there was nothing much to report. Carers felt that they could call more reviews if necessary. The drain on resources was also mentioned, with the concern that the money spent on so many meetings would adversely affect the recruitment of carers and the capacity for making new links.

Medical Assessments

What sort of reports are obtained, and for whom?

Under the Act, before a child is accommodated (that is, placed for 24 hours or more) on a family link service, the responsible authority must:

'(a) ensure that arrangements are made for the child to be examined by a registered medical practitioner, and

(b) require the practitioner who has carried out the examination to make a written assessment of the state of health of the child and his need for health care unless the child has been so examined and such assessment has been made within a period of three months immediately preceding the placement.'

(DH 1991 Family Placement Regulations, vol.3, p125)

Fifty-nine per cent of respondents in the national survey were not obtaining special medical reports and relied solely on information from parents. Of the remainder, 22 per cent used the child's most recent medical report, 16 per cent used a report from a doctor specially for the placement and nine per cent sent a standard form to GPs to complete. In six per cent of cases, more than one of these methods was being employed to gain information.

As Table 7 (page 32) shows, only 19 per cent of respondents had obtained a medical report of some description for all of the children using their service.

Very few (11%) of the children's files examined in the six services contained a written assessment of the child's health from a medical practitioner. These were predominantly in two of the study areas (South West and Midlands) and mainly in the files of children linked since the Children Act came into force. In two areas (Northern and Wales) none of the files examined contained such an assessment. The most common form of this assessment was a written report by a consultant. One area had introduced a

Table 7: **Proportion of children within each service for whom a medical report had been obtained before the start of a placement**

Report obtained for	% services (n = 172)
All children using service	19
50-99 per cent of children using service	6
1-49 per cent of children using service	16
None of children using service	59

health questionnaire which was filled in by parents and sent to GPs for verification and comment. In the majority of cases, there was no evidence that the procedure had been repeated after the start of the placement.

In contrast to this, information from the parents' questionnaires suggests that most children are being assessed regularly, even if this information is not formally noted at the link service. Over two thirds (69 per cent) of parents said that their children were having annual medicals.

Although most files did not contain health assessments by a medical practitioner, almost three quarters of the files examined contained information on the child's health needs, which had been provided by the parents. This is backed up by findings from the carers' questionnaire: 81 per cent of carers said that they had received written information about the child's health before the start of the link. Four fifths of this group stated that this information was regularly updated.

Why were medical assessments not taking place?

Staff views about medical assessments were not examined in the national survey. Some respondents made a point of commenting, however, that the requirement was not entirely appropriate. For example:

'For respite placements, a yearly health statement has little value, when many of the children are regularly seen by consultants, and parents are usually best placed to evaluate their own child's health needs.'

In the course of the interviews, staff in the six services visited explained the planned or existing procedures for obtaining medical assessments. The most common format was to obtain a copy of the latest school medical (three areas). Two services had specially designed forms which were being sent to GPs/consultants. The sixth service was following Child Minding Regulations for its link service and therefore had not made any specific plans to meet this requirement (although this particular service did have written reports in nearly half of the children's files examined). It appears that these procedures were, for the most part, still in their early stages which could explain the absence of written assessments on most of the files examined, as noted above. Moreover, not all files were looked at; it could be that there was a greater proportion of reports overall than the evidence from the sample of files suggests.

As far as staff attitudes to this Regulation were concerned, there was an even split between those respondents who accepted it and those who could not understand the reasons behind it. They argued that if child protection was behind the Regulation, then an annual statement of health would not address this issue. The same would apply if children had complex and changing medical needs – far more frequent monitoring would need to be (and was being) undertaken in these cases. Information on the health needs of children was generally being passed on anyway by consultants (where relevant) and by the parents themselves both informally and formally (in the child profile form completed by all parents before the start of a link).

Any changes in condition could also be monitored regularly at reviews. One area, while accepting the requirement for a written statement, was not planning to repeat the exercise each year: staff here thought that they might lose the goodwill of the consultants in the area who could get 'very tired of writing 180 annual medical reports when there has been little change in the child's medical status'.

Carers' and parents' views about medical assessments

All carers taking part in interviews stated that they received information on the child's health needs (in the form of a child profile) before the start of a link. All carers said that they were updated by parents on any changes, either directly as they happened or at reviews. The vast majority (nearly 90 per cent) were happy with the information that they received. A few carers commented that parents were best placed to provide this information: they knew more about their child than anyone else and it was in their interests to keep the carers well informed. Information directly from parents was also seen as being more up to date than reports from third parties.

Fewer than ten per cent of the comments related to perceived shortcomings of the system. These came from carers who felt that their current supply of information was not detailed enough or was too sporadic. They wanted more information in writing. In one area a dosage card was about to be introduced which would travel with the child between their home and the carer's home, and on which all details of medication (for example, dosage, time of last dose) would be noted. Three carers in this area welcomed the idea.

Parents were asked for their views regarding the requirements for the link service to have a regularly updated medical report on file. About two thirds of parents were happy for this to take place. Some parents thought that this was particularly important if a child had complex needs which needed monitoring. For example:

> 'They need the information, they need to know the medical conditions, to be in possession of the full facts, to be as wise as we are.'

Others thought that a written record would be useful in case they forgot any details.

About half of all the parents interviewed, however, had reservations about the new requirement. About one quarter of parents were clear that they did not want their children to have to undergo a separate medical, as they already had to go through enough:

> 'I ticked a box giving them access to medical records, which is fine. I'm not having him mauled about again.'

A similar number felt that, in many cases, they were the best source of knowledge about their child and would pass information on as necessary. A smaller number of parents commented that for medically stable children the requirement seemed less relevant.

Very few parents (four per cent) made negative comments. These included the view that the new requirement was a waste of time when they provided the information anyway, and the feeling that the new system would be an invasion of privacy.

The limit on care

How many days did children spend with carers?

The Children Act Family Placement Regulations stipulate an upper limit to the number of days a child can spend with a carer as part of a series of short-term breaks in any one year. The limit stands at 90 days, but in the six services visited in phase two of the study, the majority of children are spending much less time than this with their carers. Most areas had allocation limits set at between 28 and 50 days per year. These were largely dictated by budgetary considerations. Only one area had no maximum (the

South west, where the Family Placement Regulations were not being followed) but if the number of days went above 90 days, the placement was considered to be 'shared care' and extra monitoring by all agencies was instituted.

From the files examined, only one out of 105 children had stayed away for more than 90 days between April 1992 and March 1993. The spread of allocations is shown in Figure 3 below. Some of the children with no allocation details on file had joined the service after April 1993. For the rest, it is quite likely that many would have had to adhere to the standard allocation outlined above.

Attitudes to the 90-day limit

The 90-day limit was generally seen by staff as sensible, as long as there was a built-in flexibility to go over the limit in special cases (for example, a prolonged stay in hospital by a parent). Extra monitoring was seen as good practice in these cases. If 90 days were being requested without any particular reason, then staff would

Figure 3:   Allocated days on children's files (Apr 1992 – Mar 1993) (n = 105)

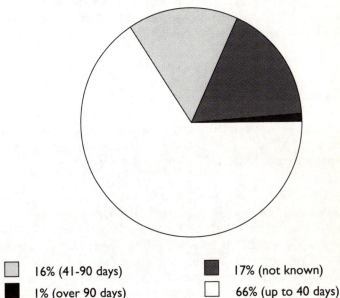

16% (41-90 days)	17% (not known)
1% (over 90 days)	66% (up to 40 days)

be concerned. However, as one member of staff pointed out, there did not appear to be any formal sanctions after this limit. If the placement was then classed as long term, the number of required reviews would actually drop to two per year instead of three.

Parents found it hard to imagine what 90 allocated days would be like, as most of them had nowhere near that amount. The idea of a limit of 90 days, however, was generally accepted as sensible. Half of the parents wanted to see some scope for flexibility, either for children with exceptionally high needs or for emergencies.

Charging for use of the service

Local authorities are now allowed to charge for the services that they provide (DH, 1989, Section 29(1)). In the national survey, two per cent of services said that they were charging all users for the periods of care provided, and 14 per cent stated that they charged some of their users (mainly those aged over 16, in receipt of their own benefit). This represents a marked increase in charging since the survey conducted by Shared Care [UK] in 1989–1990 (Orlik and others, 1991), when fewer than two per cent of children's link services reported that they were charging any users at all. The trend for charging was, however, already evident in the second Shared Care[UK] survey (Beckford and Robinson, 1993), where seven per cent of children's services were charging at least some of their users.

In four out of the six areas visited in phase two of the study, no children were being charged for use of the link service. In the South Coast service charging was universal (75 per cent of the care component of the Disabled Living Allowance), although those on Income Support were exempt and no one was refused the service if they could not afford to pay. In the Northern service, children who were over 16 and on benefit also faced a charge.

Attitudes to charging

In all areas except the South Coast, staff disagreed with the principle of universal charging. Staff of the South Coast service thought it was reasonable practice. Staff in the Northern service thought it slightly more acceptable to charge those who were over 16, as they received money of their own. The main objections to charging raised by most staff were that people might be deterred from using the service (especially if they were ambivalent about it in the first place) or simply would not be able to afford it, particularly since the cost of caring for children with disabilities is already much higher than for non-disabled children (Bennett and

Arahams, 1994). Two respondents thought that charging might cost more to administer than it raised.

Half of the parents were strongly against charging, pointing out that the costs of disability were already very high. In addition, they argued that the cost of keeping children in care would be much higher than enabling them to live at home, so parents should not be charged for the service. Parents also commented that a charge would exclude either themselves or others on a low income from using the service.

Just under half of the parents said that they would not mind paying a small charge if the service was otherwise at risk. Many of these were clear that they could not survive without the service. Provisos included the need for means testing and the view that only those over 16 who had their own money should be charged. Only three of this group of parents saw charging as positive or fair. The remainder would accept it only if it were absolutely necessary.

Parents from minority ethnic groups

Of the 105 files examined, 16 related to children from minority ethnic groups. These indicated that the implementation of the Act was generally fairly consistent with the sample as a whole. The differences were a higher proportion who had not had reviews noted in the last year (31 per cent, compared with 23 per cent of the whole sample) and a greater proportion of children with full plans (31 per cent compared with 13 per cent of the whole sample).

Twelve of the 66 parents interviewed were from minority ethnic groups. The majority (eight) spoke good English and were therefore interviewed by the project researcher. The views expressed among these parents were similar to those of the sample as a whole. The remaining four parents were interviewed by a researcher who spoke their language. In terms of the Regulations, these parents did not appear to have had very different experiences: three out of four had been involved in drawing up their child's plan and had received a copy, and had been invited to review meetings (although only two of the four had attended the reviews). There was, nevertheless, a problem with communication, particularly since neither of the two services concerned employed staff who could speak the relevant languages. For example:

> 'I would like an Asian worker to come regularly. When introductions began there was no interpreter. If my daughter was not available, I would not know what was happening' (translated).

This particular service was developing links with an Asian support group with a view to addressing this problem. This is to be welcomed, since without such communication, it is difficult to see how any partnership with parents can be achieved.

Discussion

Implementation of the Regulations is clearly causing difficulties for family link services. A recent Social Services Inspectorate report came to similar conclusions, describing implementation as 'patchy' (SSI, 1994). The services we spoke to appear to be coping with the Regulations by interpreting them loosely. This, too, is backed up by SSI findings: their report notes that in some cases, the child's assessment had been understated to the extent that parents did not even realise that it had taken place.

Deregulation is obviously not the answer – the welfare of vulnerable children would then be at risk. Unworkable regulations which are interpreted loosely are not the ideal solution either. A balancing act is needed so that children are protected by a set of realistic regulations which recognise the circumstances of short-term care. The latest Children Act Report by the Department of Health (DH, 1994a) comes to the same conclusion, calling for a balance between safeguarding the welfare of the child and maintaining the highly valued flexibility of the service. We welcome this statement and the decision to review the Regulations by issuing consultation papers (DH, 1994b, 1995). In reviewing the Regulations we hope that the points discussed below will be considered.

Full assessments and plans for children with disabilities using family link services in our study were not widespread. The SSI study mentioned above (SSI, 1994) also found that, where assessments of children were taking place, they tended to be related to one element of the services available, rather than looking at the needs of the child as a whole. This study and a recent Audit Commission report (Audit Commission, 1994) noted a shortage of multi-agency planning structures within local authorities. Without such structures, the likelihood of full assessments taking place is inevitably reduced.

The question remains as to whether a full plan for every child using short-term care services is the best use of resources. Would it be more sensible to institute full planning procedures once usage had reached a certain number of days per year, or after the first year of service use? The problem then arises that children using more than one short-term care service (for example, family-based and residential) are in danger of drifting into long-term care without anyone realising, if no overall planning mechanism exists. Thought must be given to a means of ensuring that keyworkers are available who have the time to take this overview for these children, or of establishing a coordinating panel which considers the use of all relevant services by individual children.

The reviewing frequency laid down in the Regulations is at odds with the reviewing frequency for long-term care, where only two reviews per year are required. There seems to be a consensus that two reviews per year are sufficient, with the facility to call more if necessary. It would therefore be logical to reduce the reviewing frequency to twice per year, at least for links which have been established for a year or more.

The requirement for a health assessment makes sense in a fostering context, given that child protection is often an issue and that the health needs of children in long-term care may be neglected (Parker and others, 1991). In family link services, however, the reasons for this requirement are less clear. If the concern is to keep abreast of changes in medical conditions and medication, then this could (and should) be provided throughout the year using other systems. Any changes could be passed on to the link service by consultants/GPs as necessary. One area in our study had already instituted a dosage card system to ensure that medication information was always available.

An initial visit in the early stages of a placement is important, particularly in the case of emergency placements. However, given the efforts that are put in to ensuring that all parties are happy with the link before an overnight stay takes place, an initial visit during the first stay would seem to be unnecessary and potentially disruptive. A visit within a certain number of overnight stays, combined with regular telephone contact before this, would therefore be more appropriate.

Finally, there are two loopholes in the Family Placement Regulations which are causing some confusion. The Regulations apply to stays of 24 hours or more. Children who go to their link families after school and leave the next morning could be away from home for up to five days in this situation without coming under the Regulations if the 24-hour rule is interpreted literally. The position needs to be clarified. One way forward would be to apply the Regulations for stays of 12 hours or more.

The second area of confusion is the limit on the number of days during which a child can stay away from home per year. At present this stands at 90 days (but the Department of Health consultation papers (DH, 1994b, 1995) propose to raise this to 120), after which the placement is no longer considered to be respite care. It is not clear from the Regulations, however, whether this limit applies to the use of all short-term care services combined, or each service individually. Given that previous research has shown that between 18 and 21 per cent of children in each of three local authority areas were using more than one kind of short-term care facility (Robinson and Stalker, 1989), it is important that this loophole be addressed. If a child can have 90 days in up to three facilities then it is evident that the links with parents may become extremely tenuous without any formal intervention being required.

3. Regulations for carers

Registration of carers

How were carers registered?

Under the Children Act, all carers providing short-term breaks of 24 hours or more should be registered foster carers. This involves numerous checks and a lengthy approval process. In the national survey, 85 per cent of carers providing overnight accommodation for respondents' services had been registered as foster carers. For 12 per cent, a fostering assessment had been carried out but they were registered as a 'shared carer' or 'link family'. Only two per cent of carers were registered as childminders and one per cent as volunteers. (Both these forms of registration involve fewer checks and a less stringent approval process than the foster care assessment.) Virtually all services were using only one form of registration.

Five of the six areas visited were following the foster carer approval process, re-registering carers where necessary. This is reflected in the registrations found on file. In these five areas around 90 per cent of the files examined showed that the carer had been registered specifically for short-term care using foster care procedures. The sixth area was currently registering carers specifically for short-term care, undertaking most of the same checks as for foster carers and carrying out an assessment, but not taking the application to panel. This area (in the South West) was about to introduce childminding registration for all its short-term carers.

The proportion of foster care registrations across all areas in the files examined was 70 per cent, with a further 15 per cent not following the full procedure (South West). The remaining data were not on file.

The data from carers' questionnaires back up these findings. Around three quarters of carers stated that they had been registered as foster carers and 23 per cent said that they had been registered as carers specifically for short-term care (for example, respite carers, family support workers).

What checks were undertaken?

Table 8 indicates the percentage of respondents in the national survey conducting the checks on foster carers that are required by the Family Placements Regulations of the Children Act. It is clear that examination of official documents such as birth and marriage certificates is not usual, although this is required by the Family Placement Regulations. Medical reports were obtained in most cases, and police reports in all cases.

Table 8:   The percentage of services where the foster care approval process was operational, undertaking each of the steps specified

		Percentages of services (n = 161)
1	Police check for applicants	100
2	Police check for other adults in applicant's household	100
3	Interviews with two referees	91
4	Examination of birth certificate	34
5	Examination of marriage certificate (if applicable)	52
6	Examination of naturalisation documents (if applicable)	22
7	Written medical report from a doctor	94
8	Checks with other agencies, eg NSPCC, Probation, Education	68

Police checks and references from GPs had been obtained for virtually all the carers whose files were examined. Checks with other agencies were less common (for example, social services, education, probation and NSPCC). Interviews with two referees are now a required part of the approval process. Just under two thirds of the files showed that this had taken place (in some cases up-dating existing approvals).

Reviewing and reapproving carers

The Family Placement Regulations stipulate that foster carers must be reviewed at least once a year and reapproved. In the national survey, the vast majority of respondents (89 per cent) intended to comply with this requirement, although this might not necessarily involve returning to an approval panel or re-doing any checks. Although this figure refers to intention rather than actual reviewing, it indicates that the increase in annual carer reviews noted in Beckford and Robinson (1993) from 52 per cent to 68 per cent (pre- and post- Children Act respectively) is likely to continue.

Five of the six services visited were using the Family Placement Regulations. As demonstrated in Figure 4, just over half of the files in these areas showed that the carers had been reapproved annually, as specified by the Regulations. According to data from the carers' questionnaires, the number of carers whose approval had been reviewed annually was higher: 83 per cent.

In two areas reapproval did not involve returning to the foster care panel or re-doing any checks. In one area applications went back to panel for existing carers to be registered following the Act or if there were any subsequent changes in circumstances. In the Midlands, annual reapprovals always went to panel without re-doing checks, while in London the approval panel was involved every two years, with checks being re-done every year.

Figure 4:   Frequency of carers' review noted on files (n = 75)

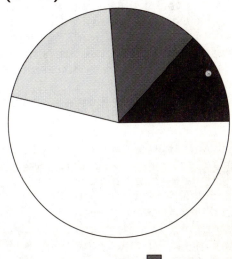

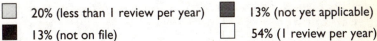

20% (less than 1 review per year)   13% (not yet applicable)

13% (not on file)   54% (1 review per year)

Attitudes to carer registration

In the six services visited the foster carer registration requirement was viewed positively by all staff. In four areas such procedures had always been carried out, with carers being registered specifically for short-term care. The fact that this was now a requirement was seen by some staff to raise the status of carers.

Staff in all areas thought that the requirement to review approvals was a good one. (All were already doing so or planning to do so). Reviews were thought to give carers the opportunity to express concerns or opinions, to plan for the future, or to withdraw in an acceptable manner if they wanted to do so. As a result, carers would feel that they were being listened to. Despite these positive attitudes, a few staff did highlight the large amount of extra work involved in meeting this requirement.

Carers taking part in interviews accepted that the foster carer registration process was necessary in order to safeguard the child. As one carer commented:

> 'I agree with it. Anyone who has close contact with disabled children should be checked out for the child's protection.'

Fewer than one in five comments on this subject were in any way negative. These were mainly concerned with the length of the process and the apparent repetition of work for those who had been registered already elsewhere. A small number of carers initially felt daunted by the prospect of the registration process but felt better once it had started.

The association with foster care did not seem to be an issue for carers. It was regarded as being a name only and did not affect their service, which was seen as quite separate from fostering. There were one or two negative comments about the inappropriate wording on some of the forms (for example, terms that applied to long-term care and not to their situation).

Carers accepted the need for reapproval as a means of safeguarding the child and reassuring the parent. They also saw the review as an opportunity to raise queries or problems, to update the service on any changes in circumstances, or to withdraw from the service. Fewer than one in five carers were either critical of or indifferent to this requirement. Some carers thought that it was not necessary, or at least not needed every year, as the service staff knew them well and were in regular contact anyway. The extra work involved for staff was also commented upon.

Over half of parents from the five services that were operating the foster care registration saw this process in a positive light. It was viewed as reassuring and a good precaution: about one in seven of parents in these five services commented that the process must be stressful for carers. On the other hand, if they were successful, this was seen as indication of their suitability as carers. One in five parents commented on the associations with fostering. A few did not like the implications of the term, suggesting that their children were 'in care'. On the whole, however, those who raised the issue felt that it was just a name and so did not matter.

Carers' documents

Who received Foster Care Agreements and Foster Placement Agreements?

Foster Care Agreements detail the responsibilities of the agency and the carer. Foster Placement Agreements detail specific responsibilities of carers for individual children. Under the Children Act, these documents should be issued to every carer. However, as Figures 5 and 6 show (page 46), services who took part in the national survey were generally either issuing them to all their carers or to none.

Both our survey and the Shared Care^{UK} survey conducted shortly after the introduction of the Children Act (Beckford and Robinson, 1993) indicated that 26 per cent of services were not issuing either of these documents to any of their carers. The lack of progress in this area is a cause for concern.

The services that were managing to issue Foster Placement Agreements were struggling with the associated requirement to review them three times per year, the aim being to ensure that the placement continues to meet the needs of the child. Only 18 per cent of all services, however, were complying with this requirement. Over half of the services were reviewing these Agreements less frequently, and one third did not have any Agreements to review.

According to the sample of files examined in the six services visited, approximately four in five carers had been issued with a Foster Care Agreement (or an equivalent document). Sixty-eight per cent of the files showed that Foster Placement Agreements (or their equivalent) had been issued for each child going to stay with the carer. A further 12 per cent of carers had received Foster Placement Agreements for at least some of the children placed with them.

The carers' postal survey produced similar figures for the Foster Care Agreement: 87 per cent of carers said that they had received

Figure 5:   Proportion of Services issuing Foster Care Agreements (n = 172)

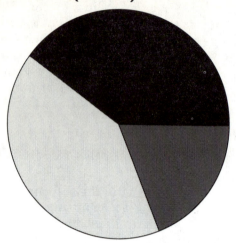

- ■ 40% (no carers (on service) receive FCA)
- ▨ 19% (some carers (on service) receive FCA)
- □ 41% (all carers (on service) receive FCA)

Figure 6:   Proportion of services issuing Foster Placement Agreements (n = 172)

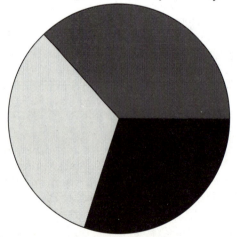

- ▨ 37% (all carers (on service) receive FPA)
- □ 33% (no carers (on service) receive FPA)
- ■ 30% (some carers (on service) receive FPA)

such a document. In the case of Foster Placement Agreements, the figure from the carers' questionnaire is higher than that found in the sample of files: 89 per cent said that they had received a document for each child placed with them giving details of the child and the planned placement. Some of the discrepancy might be explained by a slight difference in the make-up of the two samples. It could also be that some carers were referring to the child profile, in which parents give a detailed description of the child, rather than the Foster Placement Agreement. During the group interviews there was a certain amount of confusion as to whether the Placement Agreement was, at least in part, the child profile. This could have been the case in the postal survey too.

Attitudes to carers' documents

All staff in the six services visited thought that the Foster Care Agreement (outlining the respective responsibilities of agency and carer) was essential. They maintained that carers needed to know what the job involved and what was expected of them. There were, however, one or two reservations. One member of staff was concerned about the use of the same document as that issued to long-term carers: some of the content of the form was not appropriate for short-term breaks. Another staff member wondered if the document would ever be read, given the amount of paperwork the carers received.

The issuing of Foster Placement Agreements was also seen as good practice by all staff. The reservations expressed were exactly the same in content and degree as for the Foster Care Agreement.

In the group interviews, carers' reactions to the Foster Care Agreement were mainly either positive or indifferent. About two thirds of carers liked to have something in writing so that they knew where they stood and in order to formalise their relationship with the authority. Comments included:

> 'I think it's a good thing, a rule book, you know what your expectations are and what they expect from you.'

and:

> 'It's not a bad thing. If you've ever got a query, you can refer to it.'

About one third of carers either could not remember the Foster Care Agreement or did not refer to it. Those who did not refer to it thought that they could manage without it, as they worked so closely with the parent and child. This group of carers did not object, however, to receiving the document if this was a requirement. The small minority of negative comments referred to the unnecessary bureaucracy and irrelevance of some parts of the documents.

Only one third of carers felt able to comment about the Foster Placement Agreements: many could not remember having received one, although all had received a child profile at the start of the placement.

As with the Foster Care Agreement, comments were either positive or neutral. On the positive side, carers liked to have everything on paper and welcomed anything that safeguarded the child. Those who were indifferent to the document stated that they did not refer to it so it did not really affect them. Again there were a few negative comments about the cost of the extra paperwork and about the inappropriateness of some of the wording on the forms.

Preparation and training of carers

The Children Act Family Placement Regulations state that services should provide training for all their carers and meet the costs of attending such training. This issue was not investigated in great detail in the national survey, nor were details about the training provided by the six services visited generally held on individual carers' files.

Which programmes were in place?

All six areas visited provided preparation for carers before they were approved, some of them more formally and extensively than others. In four areas there were specific training sessions, three of which were exclusively for carers preparing to be approved. These were held in concentrated blocks of six to eight weeks. The fourth area offered combined training sessions for carers at all levels of involvement in the service, from 'pre-approval' candidates through to experienced carers. These same four areas also offered on-going training for carers once they had been approved.

The remaining two areas (South Coast and South West) offered one-to-one preparation for all their potential carers. This may have been dictated, to an extent, by the fact that both these services operated in large rural areas where group training sessions would have been problematic. No on-going training was mentioned by staff in these areas. In the South Coast service there were only three carers, all of whom had extensive experience from relevant professions. If other less experienced carers were taken on, then more training would be offered.

Training specifically relating to the Children Act was generally incorporated into existing programmes. Relevant information and explanations were also contained in the documents issued to carers by each service.

Recruitment of carers

Had the number of carers changed since the introduction of the Children Act?

In the national survey, just over one in three respondents (37 per cent) thought that the number of carers offering overnight stays for their service had increased since the introduction of the Children Act. Around half of these services had invested resources to recruit more carers. Others cited natural growth, the fact that they had only been set up recently, or a higher awareness of their service as being the reasons for the increase in number of carers.

Fifty-three per cent of services had noted no increase in the number of carers on their books offering overnight stays, and a further nine per cent had actually lost carers since the introduction of the Children Act. The absence of growth was mainly attributed to lack of resources available to invest in recruitment, exacerbated in some cases by the new workload associated with implementing the Children Act.

The majority of respondents (88 per cent) thought that the number of carers from minority ethnic groups had not changed since the introduction of the Children Act, either because this number reflected the general population, or because extra resources had not been invested and workloads were constraining any recruitment activity. Seven per cent of services had witnessed an increase in the number of carers from minority ethnic groups, attributed to greater resources being made available and/or specific recruitment drives.

According to records at the six services visited, the number of carers had increased in two areas, from 113 to 120, and from 31 to 46. In the latter case, staff thought that the increase was due to natural growth as the scheme was a fairly new one. Two services had witnessed no change since the introduction of the Children Act, and one service had lost a few carers (51 down to 45). One service had only been operating since the introduction of the Children Act, so the question did not apply (South Coast).

How were carers recruited?

The most common form of recruitment in all services visited was word of mouth. In addition, most services advertised in a variety of media (local papers/radio or leaflets and posters in public places). The problem, according to staff in three services, was not lack of interest, but a lack of resources to deal with that interest. In one of these services, leaflets and posters were being deliberately withheld as the coordinator was unable to deal with the likely response, in terms of the hours which would be involved in the preparation and assessment of potential carers. Staff in another service felt able only to recruit enough staff to replace those who left, as the service could not support any more than the current number of carers. This problem existed before the introduction of the Children Act: in the first Shared Care[UK] survey, coordinators were unable to invest enough time in following up enquiries from potential carers (Orlik and others, 1991). The Children Act requirements have obviously not alleviated the situation.

Two of the three areas serving minority ethnic populations thought that they had not been very successful in recruiting carers from these groups. Various attempts had been made to appoint appropriate staff who could undertake this recruitment as well as support carers once they had joined the service. A variety of factors had caused these initiatives to fail and the services were now looking at new ways forward. The third service was reasonably happy with its recruitment procedures and had in fact increased the proportion of carers from minority ethnic groups from 14 to 29 per cent of all its carers.

Carers from minority ethnic groups

Fourteen of the 90 carers' files examined related to carers from minority ethnic groups. No significant differences were noted with regard to the implementation of the Regulations for this group.

Eleven of the 69 carers interviewed were from minority ethnic groups. Most of them (nine) spoke good English and were therefore interviewed by the project researchers. The remaining two were interviewed by another researcher who spoke their language. One of these carers had extensive involvement with the service (for example, consulted by staff, attended reviews, received carers' documents, and a social worker had visited the child in placement). The other carer, in contrast, had had none of this involvement, although an invitation to attend reviews had been given. This carer highlighted communication difficulties as the main source of the problem and expressed the need for an Asian worker:

'so I can exchange my views in my own language.' (translated)

The other carer endorsed this, stating that in this way a

'better relationship can be built between the three parties: carer, social worker and the family who uses the service.' (translated)

In three areas the proportion of carers from minority ethnic groups had increased either slightly or substantially from 19 to 20 per cent, six to eight per cent, and 14 to 29 per cent respectively of all carers on the service. In the other three areas, there was no significant minority ethnic population.

Discussion

The Regulations surrounding issues of carer approvals and reviews are less controversial than those that directly affect children and their families. The carers we spoke to accepted the new requirements as being in the interests of the child.

Carers' reactions to the requirements seemed to be largely dependent on the feelings of goodwill and loyalty towards the service which had developed as a result of the efforts of the link service staff. There is a danger, however, that the amount of time and energy which staff can devote to supporting carers will be severely curtailed if excessive workloads are not addressed.

Our study highlighted a slowing down in recruitment and making new links. Staff were not happy about the amount of support that they could provide for carers. There were also fears that carers might leave as a result of new registration and reviewing requirements. Although the findings from the six services in phase two of the study indicate that this has not happened, the concerns should not be ignored. The carers form the backbone of the service and their contributions are vital. The time and energy required to recruit and support them must be included in the equation if high quality services are to be achieved.

4. Overview

Overall effects

Findings from the national survey

The results from the postal survey clearly indicate that the requirements of the Children Act are causing problems for link service coordinators. Evidence from the survey suggests that the increased workload that the Family Placement Regulations entail could mean that fewer children receive the service. The number of users in over half of the services taking part had remained static since the introduction of the Children Act. In a further eight per cent of services, numbers of users had fallen. The fact that a standstill or decline was reported in nearly two out of three services is even more alarming in the light of the previous 50 per cent growth in the overall number of children using the services noted between 1990 and 1992 (Beckford and Robinson, 1993).

In addition, 22 per cent of respondents thought that the support they provided to carers had decreased since the Act's introduction. Fifteen per cent thought some long-standing carers had left because of the Family Placement Regulations and another seven per cent thought some might leave soon.

Many social workers were unhappy about the legislation's effects on their service. They complained that lack of resources and increased workloads left little time for recruiting and supporting carers and making new links. One coordinator said:

'All assessments now take at least 50 hours to complete; our scheme is underfunded for the new legislation. We have stopped making any new links until we receive more funding for the carers' budget and coordinator hours.'

Respondents also feared that the formality of the Regulations could be off-putting for parents and carers, making them feel less in control. This threat to a sense of partnership contradicts one of the Act's main tenets. One respondent said:

> 'I feel the requirements of the Children Act have placed unnecessary burdens on carers, workers and users. This detracts from family-based respite care by making arrangements more inflexible and introducing unnecessary 'red tape'. Existing good practice may well be eroded by such formality and form-filling.'

The experiences in the six services visited

The number of children using the service had remained the same since the introduction of the Children Act in three of the six services visited (one of these had only been operating since the Act was introduced). A fourth service had witnessed a slight increase. In two out of the six services, the numbers had risen from 41 to 70, and 37 to 56 respectively.

Before considering the Family Placement Regulations in detail, staff were asked for their views on the overall effects of the Children Act, both positive and negative. In four of the six services, staff commented on the extra workload and paperwork which the Regulations entailed. In one service, this was preventing the member of staff from following up carer inquiries. This respondent was also reluctant to make new links as she did not have the time to support them.

In the remaining two services, one had only been operating since the Children Act and therefore the member of staff could not comment on any changes since before the Act. The workload of the Act would, however, put a limit on the number of new links which could be made. In the other service, the Regulations were not being followed, so again no comments were made on the overall impact of the Children Act.

On the positive side, the reviewing requirement (but not its frequency) was seen to be a good introduction, with the reservation that it should not become over-formalised.

Staff reported that some parents had initially had some fears about the use of the term 'accommodation' and its associations with being 'in care'. Staff had managed to allay these anxieties by handling the requirements sensitively and explaining the reasons behind them.

Staff thought that there had been very little adverse reaction from carers, mainly because they had worked hard to maintain support for the carers, had explained the requirements in detail and had kept everything 'light hearted'. Long-standing carers had accepted re-registration 'in the interests of the child'.

At a later stage in the interview, staff were asked in further detail about the support they provided for their carers. Few respondents were happy with the support that could be given to carers. Staff in two of the six services felt that they were not offering enough support and only visited carers if they received a specific request. Staff in the remaining three services felt that they were managing to provide enough support but only just, and that they would not be able to cope if the Children Act were to be interpreted literally or if they had any more carers.

All staff were putting a great deal of effort into supporting their carers. Many reported that this would not be possible without a 'flexible' attitude to working hours which was inevitably taking its toll on individual staff.

The efforts made by staff were reflected in both carers' and parents' views. Virtually all the carers interviewed (except one) were happy with the support and contact they had from link staff. They were 'always there if you need them' or 'only a phone call away'. A few carers mentioned that link staff seemed overwhelmed with paperwork since the Children Act was implemen- ted, and so had less time for informal visits. These respondents were not complaining: they felt, as did all carers, a great deal of loyalty towards and sympathy with the link staff. Carers were highly satisfied with the link staff and full of praise for them, especially for the fact that they were always ready to listen and help and that nothing was too much trouble.

The majority of parents interviewed (nearly three quarters) stated that they were satisfied with the amount of support from, or contact with, link staff (or social workers where relevant). A few of these parents had previously been unhappy due to bad experiences with individual staff, or non-existence of support, but this had now changed. Very few of the remaining parents were actually dissatisfied with their service.

In summary then, it appears that staff had worked hard to ensure that carers and parents were not adversely affected by any of the changes. The results of this were reflected in carers' and parents' positive views.

The way forward

Experiences in the six services visited

At the end of their interviews, staff were asked for their views on what, if anything, was needed to ensure effective implementation of the Children Act for family-based short-term care. Respondents generally welcomed the Act, pointing out that it had raised the profile of children with disabilities and that it had introduced some necessary guidelines to work within. Respondents feared, however, that if the guidelines, however good, were allowed to take over, then there was a risk of losing the positive elements of family link services, such as the partnership with parents, the flexibility and personal contact. The majority mentioned that there was a need to differentiate between long-term foster care and short-term breaks. In some cases, the Family Placement Regulations were thought to be more appropriate for foster care (for example, the visit during the first overnight stay).

Suggestions of things that might increase the effectiveness of the Children Act mainly related to a general loosening of the Family Placement Regulations. For example, reviews could be less frequent, and the first visit could be delayed slightly. Finally, staff hoped that more resources could be devoted both to implementing the Regulations and to promoting joint working with other agencies or departments. The call for resources was echoed in the parent and carer interviews. Carers thought that there should be more link staff, and parents thought that more money was needed to put the Regulations into practice and to offer the service to more parents.

Ultimately, however, staff were pragmatic about what could be achieved within ever-shrinking budgets:

'(The Act) has got to be realistic to be workable. We know we're not going to get more resources to run the scheme. To follow the full requirements is unrealistic, but we don't want to lose the positive parts of the Act.'

A middle way was clearly being called for by link staff.

5. Conclusions and recommendations

Prior to the implementation of the Children Act, there was wide variation in the practices of family link services, in particular regarding the status of carers and the monitoring of placements.

The Family Placement Regulations introduced by the Children Act have increased standardisation in both these areas. By giving carers a clear status as foster carers, services have generally gained a more central position within local authorities. This, in combination with the classification of children with disabilities as 'children in need', has meant that the profile of children with disabilities has risen. Other positive features, such as written agreements with parents and a structured system for reviewing placements, have also been introduced.

Although there were initial concerns that carers would not want to be seen as foster carers, this has been much less of an issue than the application of the Family Placement Regulations. The welfare of the child must be paramount and the Regulations are designed with this in mind. Many family link services, however, cannot cope with the increased workload which the Act entails. A significant amount of the legislation is not therefore being implemented, a situation that is unlikely to change unless action is taken.

In August 1994, the Department of Health issued a consultation paper (DH, 1994b) which proposed the relaxing of the current Regulations concerning initial visits, health assessments and reviews. This document suggested the following amendments:

1. That the 90-day limit on the amount of time a child may spend with a carer each year should be increased to a total of 120 days per year, in order to reduce the level of administrative monitoring.
2. To remove the annual nature of placements so that reviews are required after four weeks, three months and at six-monthly intervals thereafter.

3. To allow some discretion in the timing of the first visit to a child in placement.
4. To remove the requirement to have a medical examination and a written assessment of health prior to placement and to replace it with guidance stating that good practice will involve collecting information from the child's parents and GP to ensure that short-term carers have adequate information about the child's health care needs. The requirement for an annual health assessment would also be removed.

A further consultation paper was issued in April 1995 (DH, 1995a). The primary function of this was to propose ways in which fostering duties could be undertaken by profit-making organisations. It also proposed three additional points in relation to family-based short-term care. First, that the number of reviews in the first year be reduced from three to two, with the second review occurring after six months rather than three months, but with the review after four weeks being retained.

Second, the Department made a specific proposal about the timing of the first visit: that it should take place within two weeks of the first day of placement. The Department also invited responses on the practicality of this.

Third, with regard to health assessments, the Department proposed to remove the requirement to verify with the child's GP any information about the child's health which had been collected from parents, but suggest that this be done 'where appropriate'. The requirement for an initial health assessment would remain, but this would not need to be repeated annually.

In view of the research findings, most of the proposals put forward by both consultation papers are welcome. However, the proposal that the 90-day limit be increased to 120 days per year is not acceptable. There was no evidence from the research that the limit of 90 days was a source of difficulty for either families or social workers. Indeed, most of the children were receiving much less care per year through family links than the 90-day limit. As it has never been made clear what steps should be taken to safeguard the welfare of children if this ceiling is exceeded, creating a new limit of 120 days seems unnecessary and likely to increase the risk of children drifting into long-term care.

The proposal to remove the annual nature of placements by treating them as continuous after the first year is positive, bearing in mind the high levels of non-compliance with the requirement to conduct reviews three times per year, every year. It seems likely that a requirement to review every six months will be viewed as sensible by social workers and carers alike. However, the need for a review after four weeks is more questionable, especially if a child has had few overnight stays with a short-term carer. As with the proposal to allow discretion relating to initial visits to a child in placement, one way forward would be to give social workers more discretion within a time limit, so that the first review has to be carried out within three months or seven overnight stays, whichever is the sooner.

In order for social workers to be able to assess the child's reactions to the placement and feed this information into a review, it would be necessary to ensure that the placement visit has been made prior to the first review. In practice, the requirement to visit within two weeks of the child's first overnight stay, as suggested by the second consultation paper, may still be too rigid. The child may well not go to stay with the link family for a second time during these two weeks, in which case the social worker would still have to visit during the first overnight stay. More flexibility is needed. Hence, revised Guidance could read as follows:

'There should be a logical pattern in the monitoring of placements whereby an initial placement visit always takes place prior to the first review meeting and in all cases the review should be within three months of the first stay.'

Moreover, some discretion in relation to long-term arrangements would also be helpful. Thus additional Guidance on this read:

'Consideration should also be given to having annual reviews after five years of stable care arrangements, with the proviso that any interested party can call a review at any time.'

The proposal concerning health assessments seems appropriate and reflects current good practice, with one exception: although the Guidance stresses the importance of regular updates in writing to carers to ensure that drug and treatment information is accurate at all times, it is unfortunate that there is no actual requirement for these changes to be verified by the child's GP. This is particularly important for children with complex health care needs or progressive conditions.

Unfortunately, the consultation paper does not cover a number of other issues that were raised by the research. This includes the issue of **plans** for children.

In principle, social workers thought that plans were a good idea for the children they were placing, especially for those who were 'heavy users' (those away from home for more than 90 days per year) of the service. However, difficulties have emerged in relation to resources. With less than half of the children involved in these services having an allocated social worker, questions about who is responsible for drawing up a plan need to be answered. Social workers who run family link schemes think it is neither appropriate nor feasible for them to undertake this task. Certainly, if full child care plans which include plans for health and education provision are to be made available for all children, a substantial increase in resources would be required.

It is questionable whether this is the best use of limited resources, however. We suggest that a simpler plan covering only the arrangements of the link placement should suffice for children who are not heavy users of the service, at least for the first year of use. Thereafter, a fuller plan could be drawn up. Very regular users should have allocated key workers, whose responsibility it would be to ensure that the children are appropriately catered for by the existing pattern of care.

Another fundamental issue is associated with the **application of the Regulations**. Currently the Regulations only apply if a child has a stay of 24 hours or more with a carer.

However, many children have weekday placements which entail them going to their link families after school, staying overnight and then leaving the next morning for school. At present this pattern could be repeated for up to five nights without the Family Placement Regulations being applied. In order to remove the confusion over whether an overnight stay of less than 24 hours triggers the Family Placement Regulations, we recommend that the Regulations should apply for stays of 12 hours or more.

Moreover, the wording of Regulation 13 which defines short-term placements as occurring at the same place, within one year, for no more than four weeks at a time or 90 days in total per year, means that children may be receiving care in more than one setting and may receive up to 90 days of care in each. Given that previous research by Robinson and Stalker (1989) revealed that between 18 and 21 per cent of children were using two or more short-term care services, it is important that steps are taken to ensure children receive as much consistent care as possible. The wording of the most recent consultation paper (DH, 1995) remains ambiguous, highlighting only that certain Regulations would not apply if a child is accommodated in more than one place. Guidance needs to be clearer, stating that those children who require more than 90 days care should receive it all from the same source and, where this is not possible, in no more than **two** different settings.

Similarly, there are currently children over eight years of age who receive day care but who are not protected either by these Regulations or by the Childminding Regulations. One long-term solution would be to make both sets of Regulations more consistent and complementary. For example, by:

- putting the same emphasis on health and safety issues for foster parents as currently applies to childminders;
- carrying out a more rigorous approval procedure for child-minders;
- stating exactly when one set of Regulations ceases to apply and the other comes into force.

The proposals contained in the recent Department of Health consultation documents are likely to be published as revised Guidance in the autumn of 1995. If implemented, they will do much to relieve the burden of bureaucracy on social workers and should, in turn, facilitate some expansion in services. However, we regard any revision in the Regulations or Guidance as an opportunity to remove the loopholes that we have identified. To this end, we hope that policy makers will be willing to amend their proposals to encompass more safeguards for children with disabilities and their families.

Two key principles of the Children Act are to regard the welfare of the child as paramount and to provide support for families with children in need. The Act also highlights the need to work in partnership with parents. Family link services exemplify these principles and can act as good models for service developments with other groups of children. It is therefore important that such services do not collapse under the strain of the bureaucracy required by the Act.

Postscript

Just as this book was going to press, the Department of Health issued its revised Regulations and Guidance for the short-term placement of children (DH, 1995b). We thought it important to bring the reader up to date with the final amendments, although our comments are, by necessity, very brief.

First, the amended reviewing requirements state that the first review should take place within three months of the start of a placement, and that subsequent reviews should take place at intervals of no less than six months.

Second, the timing of the first visit has been changed: it must now take place within seven placement days or before the first review (whichever is the sooner).

Third, regarding health assessments, the Department has made no amendments to the contents of its second consultation paper on this subject (DH, 1995a). There is now a requirement for an initial health examination and assessment, but no requirement for this to be repeated annually. The Guidance comments on the importance of ensuring that changes in medication or therapeutic treatment are noted in writing.

The amendments to the visiting and reviewing requirements are most welcome and should be acceptable to practitioners, carers and parents. The amendment regarding health assessment also seems to reflect good practice, although it is unfortunate that there is no actual requirement to verify any changes in medication or treatment with the child's GP before providing the short-term carers with updated information.

The 90-day limit has been increased to 120 days, as proposed in the second consultation paper. Our previous concerns on this matter, outlined in our conclusions, therefore remain unchanged.

The amendments contain no reference to various other points which were raised in our response to the Department's consultation papers. We continue to have reservations regarding the unamended requirement for full child care plans and remain concerned that certain loopholes have not been addressed (such as the 24-hour trigger for applying the Family Placement Regulations, the lack of specific regulations for multiple placements and the lack of a regulatory framework for children over eight receiving day care). Our comments on these issues are discussed fully in Chapter 5.

Although certain crucial concerns have not yet been addressed, we welcome the positive amendments contained in the revised Regulations and Guidance.

References

Aldgate J, Bradley M and Hawley D (forthcoming) *The use of short term breaks in the prevention of long term family breakdown.* Final report to the Department of Health, University of Oxford

Audit Commission (1994) *Seen but not heard. Co-ordinating child health and social services for children in need.* HMSO

Beckford, V and Robinson, C (1993) *Consolidation or change? A second survey of family based respite care services in the United Kingdom.* University of Bristol: Norah Fry Research Centre

Bennett, F and Abrahams, C (1994) *Unequal Opportunities – children with disabilities speak out.* NCH Action for Children

Department of Health (1977) *The NHS Act 1977.* HMSO

Department of Health (1989) *The Children Act 1989.* HMSO

Department of Health (1991) *The Children Act 1989. Guidance and Regulations Vol 3, Family Placements.* HMSO

Department of Health (1994a) *Children Act Report 1993.* HMSO

Department of Health (1994b) *Consultation Paper: Children Act 1989: Short term placement (respite care) of children.* August 1994.

Department of Health (1995a) *Consultation about the delegation of fostering duties to profit-making organisations and the easement of respite care regulations.* Lassl(95)4. April 1995.

Department of Health (1995b) *Amended Regulations and Guidance for Respite Care; series of short-term placements of children* (LAC(95)14), August 1995.

Neary, V (1991) 'Mrs Brown's bad days', *Inside Community Care* 26 September 1991

Orlik, C, Robinson, C and Russell, O (1991) *A survey of family based respite care schemes in the United Kingdom.* University of Bristol: Norah Fry Research Centre

Parker R and others (1991) *Looking after children: assessing outcomes in child care.* HMSO

Robinson, C and Macadam, M (1993) 'The effects of the Children Act 1989 on short-term breaks for disabled children', *Social Care Research Findings, 32*. Joseph Rowntree Foundation

Robinson, C and Stalker, K (1989) *Time for a break. An interim report to the Department of Health*. Norah Fry Research Centre

Robinson, C and Stalker, K (1990) *Respite Care: the consumer's view*. 2nd Interim Report to the Department of Health. Norah Fry Research Centre

Robinson, C and Stalker, K (1991) *Respite care: summaries and suggestions. Final Report to the Department of Health*. Norah Fry Research Centre

Robinson, C, Weston, C and Minkes, J (1994) *Assessing quality in services to disabled children under the Children Act (1989)*. Norah Fry Research Centre

Social Services Inspectorate (1994) *Services to disabled children and their families*. HMSO

Index

Entries are arranged in letter–by–letter order (hyphens and spaces between words are ignored).

A
areas of deprivation 11
Asians 37–38, 50–51
Audit Commission Report 38

C
carers
 recruitment 49–52
 registration 4, 9, 13, 41–45, 53
 training/support 9, 23, 48–49, 54
 views of child care plans 28–31, 58–59
 views of Family Placement Regulations 1–4, 9, 44, 52–54
charging 7, 9, 13, 36–37
child care legislation *see* legislation on child care
child care plans 1–3, 9, 13, 19–23, 37–39, 58–59, 62
 carer's views 28–31, 58–59
 parents' views 22–23, 28–31
 reviews 2–3, 26–31, 37, 53, 56–58, 61
 social worker's views 22, 28–31, 58–59
childminders 41
Child Minding Regulations 33, 59–60
child profiles 33, 47–48

Children Act (1989) 6–7, 41, 45, 60
 impact 1, 7–9, 42–43, 45, 49, 56
 staff views 53–55
 see also Family Placement Regulations
Children Act (1989) Regulations and Guidance 4
Children Act Report 38
'children in need' *see* children with disabilities
children's involvement 13, 28–30, 58
children's views 20
children with disabilities 6–7, 56
community teams 16
consultation 9

D
day care 8
days with carers 34–36, 39–40
Department of Health 8
Department of Health consultation papers 5, 56–57
Disabled Living Allowance 36
drift in care 22, 38–39

E
eligibility for family link
        services 11, 13, 16–17
emergency foster placements
        25, 39

F
family breakdown 8
family link services 7–9, 62
    demand 7
    eligibility for 11, 13, 16–17
Family Placement Regulations
        1, 31, 34, 42, 48, 55–62
    drawbacks 5, 52–53, 55,
        59–62
    impact 14, 21, 38–40, 52–60
    revision of 61–62
    study on impact 8–18
    views of carers 1–4, 9, 44,
        51–54
    views of parents 1–4, 9,
        44–45, 52–53
    views of social workers 1–4,
        24–25, 44, 52–55
Foster Care Agreements
        45–48, 51
foster carers
    registration 4, 41–45
    reviews 42–43, 53
fostering assessment *see* foster
        carers, registration
Foster Placement Agreements
        20, 45–47
    views 47–48, 51
funding 16, 34, 52, 55

G
GPs 4, 32–33, 42

H
health 31–34

health assessments 3–4, 39,
        57–58, 61
    see also medical reports
health service units 7
home-based care 8

I
Income Support 36
initial visits 2, 23–26, 39, 57,
        61
interviews 1, 13–15, 17, 44, 47
introductory stays 2, 25

J
Joseph Rowntree Foundation 8

K
key workers *see* social workers

L
language 14, 37, 50–51
legislation on child care, 6–7
    see also Children Act (1989);
        Family Placement
        Regulations
length of stay 34–36, 39–40,
        59, 62
link placement agreements 2,
        20
local authorities 16
long-term care 6, 36
low income groups 9

M
medical reports
    on carers 42
    on children 3–4, 31–34
    see also health assessments
minority ethnic groups 9, 11,
        14, 17, 37–38, 49–51
multiple placements 38–40,
        59, 62

N

National Association for Family Based Respite Care *see* Shared Care UK

National Health Service Act (1977) 6

ninety-day limit 5, 34–36, 56–59, 61

Norah Fry Research Centre 8, 11

O

Office of Population Censuses and Surveys 7

overnight stays, definition 39

P

parental consultation 20–21, 29, 54, 60

parent/carer communication 4, 23, 26, 30, 33, 47, 50–51

parents
views of child care plans 22–23, 28–31
views of Family Placement Regulations 1–4, 9, 44–45, 52–53

police reports 42

postal survey 1, 11, 17, 21, 45, 47, 52
see also questionnaires

profit-making organisations 57

Q

questionnaires 11, 15, 21, 24, 26–27, 41, 43
see also postal survey

R

registration of carers 4

residential care 7–8

reviews *see* child care plans, reviews

S

service coordinators 11, 20, 52

service level agreements 16

shared care 35

Shared Care^{UK} 7, 11

Shared Care^{UK} surveys 21, 36, 45, 50

short-term care 1, 6, 8, 59

social services departments 7

Social Services Inspectorate Report 38

social workers 2, 13, 16, 20–21, 39
views of child care plans 22, 28–31, 58–59
views of Family Placement Regulations 1–4, 24–25, 44, 52–55
visits 23–26
workload 21–22, 28, 49–50, 52–54, 56, 58–59

special schools 16

survey profile 9–18

T

time with carers 34–36, 39–40

twenty-four hour rule 1–2, 5, 19, 39, 59, 62

V

visits 2, 23–26, 58
initial 2, 23–25, 39, 57, 61

voluntary agencies 7, 11, 16, 21, 25

W

workload *see* social workers, workload

Publications

Recent works include:

Balancing the Act

Social Work and Assessment with Adolescents

With Equal Concern...

Good Practice in Sex Education: A sourcebook for schools

Rebuilding Families After Abuse

The Silent Minority

Schools' SEN Policies Pack

Child and Family Support and Protection

Safe to Let Out?

It's Your Meeting!

A Sense of Security

The Bureau also publishes a quarterly journal, *Children & Society* – subscription rates are available on request.

For further information or a catalogue please contact:
Book Sales, National Children's Bureau, 8 Wakley Street,
London EC1V 7QE
Tel: 0171 843 6029   Fax: 0171 278 9512

Becoming a member

The National Children's Bureau offers an extensive Library and Information Service – probably the largest child care information resource in the UK. We also run a comprehensive programme of conferences and seminars, and publish a wide range of books, leaflets and resource packs. In addition, the Bureau gives members the opportunity to tap into an influential network of professionals who care about children, helping to set the agenda for the nineties and beyond.

Membership of the National Children's Bureau provides you with:

- a quarterly mailing containing:
  - *Children UK*: the Bureau's journal
  - *Highlights:* briefing papers containing summaries of research findings and recent reports of legislation on relevant issues;
- access to the library and information service including databases, books, journals and periodicals;
- first access to the findings of our research and development projects;
- advance notice of our extensive programme of conferences and seminars throughout the country and concessionary prices;
- concessionary prices and advance details for Bureau publications.

The National Children's Bureau can support you in the day to day task of meeting the needs of children and young people. For further details please contact Jane Lewis, Membership Marketing Coordinator, National Children's Bureau, 8 Wakley Street, London EC1V 7QE or call 0171 843 6047 for further information.